Measuring the Impact of the Built Environment on Health, Wellbeing, and Performance

This book reveals how subjective and objective data gathered by innovative methods of measurement give us the ability to quantify stress, health, performance, and wellbeing outcomes in different built environments. Design interventions informed by these measures, along with innovative integrated building materials, can shape the character of built environments for better health, productivity, and performance. These measures can help employers and managers calculate the return on investment (ROI) of various design interventions.

Areas of inquiry in health and the built environment are discussed in three parts: Part 1 – Fundamentals: Human, Environment, and Material Measures for Health and Wellbeing; Part 2 – Methods: Measurement Techniques, Tools, and Methods for Health and Wellbeing; and Part 3 – Applications: Case Studies and Future Directions. The rapid pace of technical innovation and entrepreneurship by interdisciplinary research teams in health and the built environment has created a need for more publications such as this book, which discuss latest tools and methods of measuring the effects of the built environment on human physiology and psychology. Emerging tools and techniques are introduced for this field of built environment design, including virtual reality immersive environments and fisheye lens photograph simulations for human wellbeing impact measures integral to the design process. The potentials and limitations of bio-responsive material systems and integrated sensing devices with wearable technologies linked to the Internet of Things are discussed in relation to human wellbeing performance improvements.

The book provides both the foundational knowledge and fundamentals for characterizing human health and wellbeing in the built environment as well as emerging trends and design research methods for innovations in this field. It will be of interest to researchers, educators, and students of architecture, interior design, and integrative medicine, as well as professionals working in health and the built environment.

Altaf Engineer is an architect and Associate Professor at the School of Architecture and University of Arizona Institute on Place, Wellbeing, and

Performance (UA IPWP) – an interdisciplinary institute at the University of Arizona that links expertise of the UA College of Medicine – Tucson, the Arizona Center for Integrative Medicine (AzCIM), and the UA College of Architecture, Planning, and Landscape Architecture (CAPLA). Altaf has expertise in using wearable devices for measuring sleep, stress, activity, and light. He is Chair of the Master of Science in Architecture Health and Built Environment degree at the UA College of Architecture, Planning, and Landscape Architecture (CAPLA).

Aletheia Ida is an architect, designer, and technologist. She has over 15 years of experience in professional architecture practice and is fluent in building performance analytics. She holds a PhD in Architectural Sciences from the Center for Architecture, Science, and Ecology at Rensselaer Polytechnic Institute in New York. Aletheia develops interdisciplinary design theory to inform applied research in emerging building technologies with an emphasis on environmental performance, material innovations, and human wellbeing.

Wooyoung Jung is an architectural engineer and scientist, and Assistant Professor in the Department of Civil and Architectural Engineering and Mechanics at the University of Arizona, Tucson, Arizona. He has a holistic professional career, dedicated to the building sector, ranging from a practitioner in the construction industry to a researcher in academia and a couple of the Department of Energy-funded national laboratories.

Esther M. Sternberg is a physician and scientist, and internationally recognized pioneer in design and health and brain-immune (science of the mind-body connection). She is Research Director, Andrew Weil Center for Integrative Medicine, Founding Director of the University of Arizona's Institute on Place, Wellbeing, and Performance, founding member of the American Institute of Architects' Design and Health Leadership Group and AIA Design and Health Research Consortium. Previously NIH Senior Scientist and Section Chief (1986–2012), she has authored more than 240 scholarly articles, edited eight scholarly books, and authored three popular books including *Healing Spaces: The Science of Place and Wellbeing* (2009), which inspired the rebirth of the design and health movement 21st century style, and *Well at Work, Creating Wellbeing in Any Workspace* (2023), which brings that science into the post-COVID era.

Health and the Built Environment

Series Editor: Mohammad Gharipour

Health and the Built Environment provides a transdisciplinary overview of community, design, and health for practicing professionals and academics. Produced in a handy, accessible format and written by a range of leading international authors, this series will provide readers with a comprehensive understanding of the relationship between health and the environment. It will discuss key concepts such as restoration, healing and therapeutic environments, community health, integrated health-care systems, evidence-based design, technology, city and public health, and sustainability, along with many more.

Urban Environments and Health in the Philippines
A Retrospective on Women Street Vendors and their Spaces
Mary Anne Alabanza Akers

Measuring the Impact of the Built Environment on Health, Wellbeing, and Performance
Techniques, Methods, and Implications for Design Research
Altaf Engineer, Aletheia Ida, Wooyoung Jung and Esther M. Sternberg

For more information about this series, please visit: https://www.routledge.com/planning/series/HBE

Measuring the Impact of the Built Environment on Health, Wellbeing, and Performance

Techniques, Methods, and Implications for Design Research

Altaf Engineer, Aletheia Ida,
Wooyoung Jung, and
Esther M. Sternberg

Routledge
Taylor & Francis Group

LONDON AND NEW YORK

First published 2024
by Routledge
4 Park Square, Milton Park, Abingdon, Oxon OX14 4RN

and by Routledge
605 Third Avenue, New York, NY 10158

Routledge is an imprint of the Taylor & Francis Group, an informa business

© 2024 Altaf Engineer, Aletheia Ida, Wooyoung Jung, and Esther M. Sternberg

British Library Cataloguing-in-Publication Data
A catalogue record for this book is available from the British Library

Library of Congress Cataloging-in-Publication Data
Names: Engineer, Altaf, author. | Ida, Aletheia, author. | Jung, Wooyoung, author. | Sternberg, Esther M., author.
Title: Measuring the impact of the built environment on health, wellbeing, and performance : techniques, methods, and implications for design research / Altaf Engineer, Aletheia Ida, Wooyoung Jung and Esther Sternberg.
Description: Abingdon, Oxon ; New York, NY : Routledge, 2024. | Series: Health and the built environment | Includes bibliographical references and index. |
Identifiers: LCCN 2023055712 (print) | LCCN 2023055713 (ebook) | ISBN 9780367414818 (hardback) | ISBN 9781032746128 (paperback) | ISBN 9780367814748 (ebook)
Subjects: LCSH: Industrial hygiene--United States--Case studies. | Industrial hygiene--Research--Methodolgy. | Office buildings--Health aspects--United States--Case studies. | Built environment--Health aspects--United States--Case studies. | Architecture--Human factors--United States--Case studies. | Buildings--Environmental engineering--United States--Case studies.
Classification: LCC RC967 .E55 2024 (print) | LCC RC967 (ebook) | DDC 613.6/2--dc23/eng/20240112
LC record available at https://lccn.loc.gov/2023055712
LC ebook record available at https://lccn.loc.gov/2023055713

ISBN: 978-0-367-41481-8 (hbk)
ISBN: 978-1-032-74612-8 (pbk)
ISBN: 978-0-367-81474-8 (ebk)

DOI: 10.4324/9780367814748

Typeset in Times New Roman
by codeMantra

Contents

Figures

Abbreviations

3D	Three-Dimensional
AEC	Architecture, Engineering, and Construction
AEDL	Adaptive Environments Design Lab, University of Arizona
AIA	American Institute of Architects
ANFA	Academy of Neuroscience for Architecture
API	Application Programming Interface
ASHRAE	American Society of Heating, Refrigerating, and Air-Conditioning Engineers
ASTM	American Society for Testing and Materials
AWCIM	Andrew Weil Center for Integrative Medicine, University of Arizona College of Medicine
BENCH	Biorhythmic Evaporative-cooling Nano-teCH
BioBE	Biology and the Built Environment Center, University of Oregon
BIM	Building Information Modeling
BMS	Building Management System
BPM	Beats Per Minute
CAD	Computer-Aided Design
CDC	Centers for Disease Control and Prevention
CFRC	Carbon Fiber-Reinforced Concrete
CFRG	Carbon Fiber-Reinforced Glass
CFRP	Carbon Fiber-Reinforced Polymer
CHAOS	Cooling and Heating for Architecturally Optimized Systems, Princeton University
CMU	Concrete Masonry Units
CNC	Computer Numerical Control
CND	Carbon Nanodot
CO	Carbon Monoxide
CO_2	Carbon Dioxide
COVID-19	Coronavirus Disease 2019
DBT	Dry-Bulb Temperature
DSM-V	Diagnostic Statistical Manual Version 5

DYD	Donate Your Data
ECG	Electrocardiogram
EEG	Electroencephalogram
EPA	Environmental Protection Agency
FC	Foot-candles
FEMA	Federal Emergency Management Agency
fMRI	Function Magnetic Resonance Imaging
FT2	Square Foot
GHS	Greenhouse Gas
GSA	Government Services Administration
HBCD	Hexabromocyclododecane
HBN	Healthy Building Network
HIV	Human Immunodeficiency Virus
HPDC	Health Product Declaration Collaborative
HRV	Heart Rate Variability
HUD	Housing and Urban Development
HVAC	Heating, Ventilation, and Air-Conditioning
IAQ	Indoor Air Quality
IARPA	Intelligence Advanced Research Projects Activity
iCAMP	Interdisciplinary Consortium on Advanced Motion Performance, Baylor College of Medicine
ICD-10	International Classification of Diseases Version 10
IES	Institute for Employment Studies, United Kingdom
IoT	Internet of Things
IR	Infrared Radiation
IRB	Institutional Review Board
KT	Kieran-Timberlake
LBC	Living Building Challenge
LCA	Life Cycle Analysis
LEED	Leadership in Energy and Environmental Design
LM	Lumen
LM ATL	Lockheed Martin Advanced Technology Laboratories
LSPR	Localized Surface Plasmon Resonance
LX	Lux
MOSAIC	Multimodal Objective Sensing to Assess Individuals with Context
MRT	Mean Radiant Temperature
NAAQs	National Ambient Air Quality Standards
nm	Nanometer
NO_2	Nitrogen Dioxide
NPR	National Public Radio
O&M	Operation and Maintenance
OR	Operating Room
OSHA	Occupational Safety and Health Administration

PBT	Persistent Bioaccumulative Toxicant
PCS	Personal Comfort Systems
PET	Physiological Equivalent Temperature
PIR	Passive Infrared
PM	Particulate Matter
PM2.5	Particulate Matter Sized 2.5 Microns
PM10	Particulate Matter Sized 10 Microns
PMV	Predicted Mean Vote
ppb	Parts Per Billion
ppm	Parts Per Million
PPT	Plasmonic Photothermal
PTSD	Post-traumatic Stress Disorder
PZT	Lead Zirconium Titanate
RAAMP2	Rapid Automatic & Adaptive Model for Performance Prediction
RH	Relative Humidity
ROI	Return on Investment
SAD	Seasonal Affective Disorder
SARS-CoV-2	Severe Acute Respiratory Syndrome Coronavirus 2
SEM	Scanning Electron Microscope
SHAPE	Soundscape with Hydrogel-actuated Podium Electronic
SMART	Scanning MeAn Radiant Temperature
SMM	Sustainable Materials Management
SMMs	Shape Memory Materials
SO_2	Sulfur Dioxide
T	Temperature
TCPP	Tri-chloro-propyl-phosphate
TMY	Typical Meteorological Year
UA IPWP	University of Arizona Institute on Place, Wellbeing, and Performance
$\mu g/m^3$	Micrograms per Cubic Meter
USGBC	United States Green Building Council
UV	Ultraviolet
UVA	Ultraviolet (wavelength range: 315 nm–400 nm)
UVB	Ultraviolet (wavelength range: 280 nm–315 nm)
UVC	Ultraviolet (wavelength range: 100 nm–280 nm)
VIS	Visible
VOC	Volatile Organic Compound
VP	Virtual Patient
VR	Virtual Reality
WHO	World Health Organization

Acknowledgments

Joint Acknowledgments

We appreciate Dr. Erin Driver, University of Arizona Master of Public Health candidate and Intern at the University of Arizona Institute of Place, Wellbeing & Performance, for her invaluable help in the completion of this book. Additionally, we would like to thank former Research Assistants Dr. Sandra Bernal, Faith Stoddard, and Julia Duken for all their help and support. Our deepest thanks go to our editors at Routledge, Grace Harrison and others, for recognizing the potential in our project and ushering this book through to completion. Many thanks to Dr. Mohammad Gharipour, Editor of the overall Health and the Built Environment book series at Routledge for giving us this opportunity and advising us at the beginning of this project.

Altaf Engineer

A special thanks to my three coauthors for all their insights and collaboration on this project. Thanks to the University of Arizona College of Architecture, Planning & Landscape Architecture and School of Architecture for research funding which supported the hiring of the research assistants mentioned above.

This book would not have been possible without the support of my family. To Monica, my wife – thank you for always standing by me and for your constant support and encouragement.

Wooyoung Jung

I would like to thank my coauthors who gave me the chance to join this project. My family for their support.

Esther M. Sternberg

Thanks to the Andrew Weil Center for Integrative Medicine and to my other University of Arizona affiliations for continued support: BIO5 Institute, University of Arizona Institute on Place, Wellbeing, and Performance; the UArizona Colleges of Architecture, Planning & Landscape Architecture; Science (Department of Psychology); and Agriculture and Life Sciences (School of Nutritional Sciences and Wellness). Some of the research cited in the Introduction was funded by the US General Services Administration.

Introduction

Overview

The impacts of the built environment on health and wellbeing have always been important but were largely overlooked until the SARS-CoV-2 pandemic brought the role of the built environment on viral transmission to the forefront. At the start of the pandemic, the focus was mainly on the role of ventilation on viral transmission and the need for frequent fresh air turnover and adequate filtration. While adequate ventilation and filtration are essential, it is only the starting point for the myriad ways in which the built environment affects both physical health and emotional wellbeing. Whether one gets sick from a virus – and how sick one gets – depends on three factors: the dose of exposure, the duration of exposure, and importantly the individual's resilience. While ventilation, filtration, masking, and distancing can all help to reduce the dose and duration of exposure, they do not affect a person's resilience.

In the field of integrative medicine, the Andrew Weil Center for Integrative Medicine has identified seven domains or core areas of health that in combination help to keep people resilient: sleep, resilience (stress and relaxation responses), movement, relationships, environment (green environment and air quality), nutrition, and spirituality. If designed with these elements in mind, the built environment can help people engage in these healthy behaviors or, if not designed thoughtfully, can impede them and cause illness (Engineer et al., 2021).

There are many aspects of the built environment that can cause illness. First and foremost are the materials that are used in construction – these can off-gas harmful chemicals or over time can accumulate molds, allergens, and other disease-causing factors. Prevention of illness therefore depends on starting with nontoxic materials and attention to proper maintenance of building systems, like HVAC equipment, humidifiers, and filters, to remove toxins and prevent growth of mold and bacteria, like *Legionella* that causes Legionnaires' disease.

But beyond preventing and removing toxins and disease-causing germs, the built environment must be designed to support each of the seven domains

DOI: 10.4324/9780367814748-1

of integrative health (Sternberg, 2023). It is only in this way that the places where we spend over 90% of our waking hours can help enhance resilience. This book will outline ways in which the built environment can help to enhance sleep (bright full spectrum morning light, daytime movement, reduced daytime stress), as well as movement, relationships, nutrition, spirituality, access to nature, and views of nature.

In order to design an optimal "wellbeing" built environment, we need precise quantitative guidelines for the elements of the built environment that contribute to enhancing wellbeing. We are fortunate that we live in an era when it is possible to measure the impacts of many elements of the built environment on many aspects of health using wearable health-tracking devices, in combination with environmental sensing devices, and analyzed with big data analytics to tease apart the many interactions on both the human health side and the physical built environment side.

This book will describe state-of-the-art health and environmental tracking devices, and ways in which these data can be correlated through data analytics. Some examples are a series of studies called Wellbuilt for Wellbeing, which were carried out by the University of Arizona and the U.S. General Services Administration, using wearable health-tracking devices linked to wearable and stationary environmental monitoring of up to 11 different environmental attributes, including sound, temperature, humidity, carbon dioxide (CO_2) as well as spatial office layout. In the course of these studies, we found that persons in open office bench seating were 32% more active than those in private offices and 20% more active than those in cubicles [Lindberg et al., 2018). Furthermore, those who were more active during the day were 14% less stressed in the evening after they went home, as measured by heart rate variability. They also had better sleep quality and less fatigue the next day (Goel et al., 2021; Lee et al., 2018). Furthermore, humidity outside the 30%–60% relative humidity (RH) range – less than 30% RH or greater than 60% RH – was associated with a 25% higher stress response (Razjouyan et al., 2020). Finally, noise levels less than 35 or 40 decibels as well as noise levels greater than 45 decibels were associated with higher stress levels (Srinivasan et al., 2023). Personality also plays a role, with persons scoring high on extraversion being happier in open office settings and more focused than those scoring high on neuroticism (introverts) (Baranski et al., 2023)

In combination, these findings point to the need for many choices in office design, with a variety of types of spaces for people to gather in different sized groups for different purposes, with options for quiet heads down spaces when needed. They also indicate that individualized environments are needed to suit each individual's comfort levels for optimal wellbeing and productivity. This can include local desktop humidifiers, heated desk chairs, and circadian lighting for maximal morning sunlight via light boxes if desks are not near a window.

The chapters that follow will delve into all these aspects of human health measures, building materials, and environmental measures, including sensing data and data acquisition and measurement tools and technologies. Several case studies will be presented and finally implications for future directions in this fast growing field will be discussed. The time for creating wellbeing and healthy buildings is now – this is no longer a luxury but an imperative, and this book will provide the data and guidelines for achieving these goals!

References

Baranski, E., Lindberg, C., Gilligan, B., Fisher, J. M., Canada, K., Heerwagen, J., Kampschroer, K., Sternberg, E., & Mehl, M. R. (2023). Personality, workstation type, task focus, and happiness in the workplace. *Journal of Research in Personality*, *103*, 104337.

Engineer, A., Gualano, R. J., Crocker, R. L., Smith, J. L., Maizes, V., Weil, A., & Sternberg, E. M. (2021). An integrative health framework for wellbeing in the built environment. *Building and Environment*, *205*, 108253

Goel, R., Pham, A., Nguyen, H., Lindberg, C., Gilligan, B., Mehl, M. R., Heerwagen, J., Kampschroer, K., Sternburg, E. M., & Najafi, B. (2021). Effect of workstation type on the relationship between fatigue, physical activity, stress, and sleep. *Journal of Occupational and Environmental Medicine*, *63*(3), e103–e110.

Lee, H., Razjouyan, J., Nguyen, H. Lindburg, C., Srinivasan, K., Gilligan, B., Canada, K., Sharafkhaneh, A., Mehl, M., Currim, F., Ram, S., Lunden, M., Heerwagen, J., Kampschroer, K., Sternberg, E., & Najafi, B. (2018). Sensor-Based Sleep Quality Index (SB-SQI): A new metric to examine the association of office workstation type on stress and sleep. Preprints 2018, DOI: 10.20944/preprints201808.0457.v1

Lindberg, C. M., Srinivasan, K., Gilligan, B., Razjouyan, J., Lee, H., Najafi, B., Canada, K. J., Mehl, M. R., Currim, F., Sudha, R., Lunden, M. M., Heerwager, J. H., Kampschroer, K., & Sternberg, E. M. (2018). Effects of office workstation type on physical activity and stress. *Occupational and Environmental Medicine*, *75*(10), 689–695.

Razjouyan, J., Lee, H., Gilligan, B., Lindberg, C., Nguyen, H., Canada, K., Burton, A., Sharafkhaneh, A., Srinivasan, K., Currim, F., Ram, S., Mehl, M. R., Goebel, N., Lunden, M., Bhangar, S., Heerwagen, J., Kampschroer, K., Sternberg, E. M., & Najafi, B. (2020). Wellbuilt for wellbeing: Controlling relative humidity in the workplace matters for our health. *Indoor Air*, *30*(1), 167–179.

Srinivasan, K., Currim, F., Lindberg, C. M., Razjouyan, J., Gilligan, B., Lee, H., Canada, K. J., Coebel, N., Mehl, M. R., Lunden, M. M., Heerwagen, J., Najafi, B., Sternburg, E. M., Kampschroer. K., & Ram, S. (2023). Discovery of associative patterns between workplace sound level and physiological wellbeing using wearable devices and empirical Bayes modeling. *NPJ Digital Medicine*, *6*(1), 5.

Sternberg, E. M. (2023). *Well at work: Creating wellbeing in any workspace*. New York: Little, Brown Spark.

Part I
Fundamentals
Human, Environment, and
Material Measures for Health
and Wellbeing

1 Human Health and Wellbeing Measures

Human Health Measures

Human health refers to total emotional and physical wellbeing and can be measured by physiological, neurological, behavioral, psychological, and kinesthesiological means. When normal human health measures are disrupted, it can cause abnormalities. The ability to define what is normally observed by human health measures will help determine what is considered an abnormality. Anomalies can be indicative of an internal issue; therefore, it is important to evaluate what causes normal fluctuations versus what causes abnormal fluctuations (University of Rochester Medical Center, 2019). The definition of normal health is important to discuss before discussing possible reasons for abnormal physical and mental health, ways to measure these abnormalities, and analyzing the results for better health outcomes (Figure 1.1).

Physiological Health

Vital signs measure the human body's basic functions and can assess normal human health. Parts of human physiology include heart rate, blood pressure, body temperature, and respiration rate, and explain the way the body functions. Specifically, the normal blood pressure in adult humans is below 120 mm Hg for systolic blood pressure and below 80 mm Hg for diastolic blood pressure. One blood pressure measurement that is higher or lower than normal may not indicate a serious problem but should be monitored.

The normal heart rate in adult humans is 60–100 beats per minute (bpm). Checking the pulse measures the heart rhythm and the strength of the pulse. Normal heart rate has beats that vary naturally, but can also fluctuate based on exercise level, illness, anxiety levels, and gender. Doctors and other health-care professionals usually check a pulse by firmly pressing on arteries that are located on the side of the neck, inside the elbow, at the wrist, or in the groin.

Normal body temperature can range from 97.8°F to 99°F (36.6°C to 37.2°C). Healthy fluctuations in this temperature are due to fluid and food

DOI: 10.4324/9780367814748-3

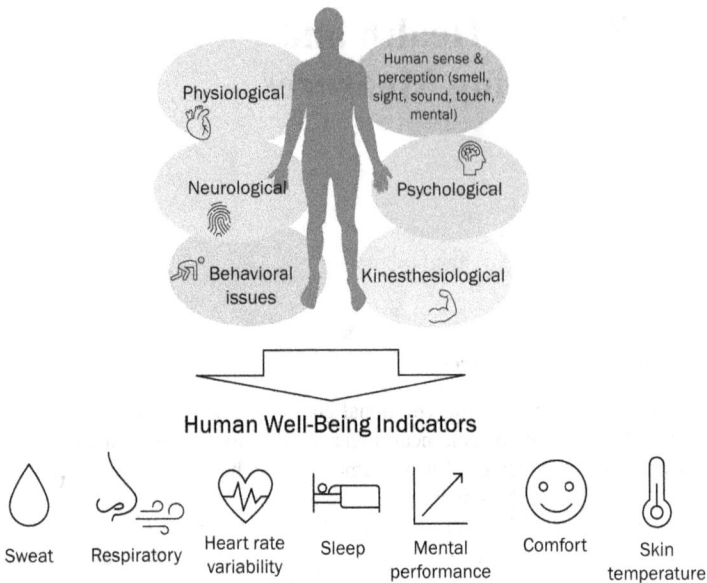

Figure 1.1 Composite Diagram: Human Figure and Related Health Measures and Characteristics.

consumption, thermoregulation, time of day, gender, and age. A person's body temperature can be checked orally, rectally, by ear, by skin, by armpit, or internally by probes that are placed in the esophagus, heart, or bladder.

Normal respiration rate is checked when a person is at rest and involves counting how many times the chest rises and falls within the minute. A normal range is from 12 to 16 breaths per minute. An increase in the number of breaths taken per minute can indicate that an individual is struggling to breathe or not getting enough oxygen (University of Rochester Medical Center, 2019).

While these conventional methods of measuring vital signs and assessing an individual's physiological health are accurate and efficient, they are limited to clinical and research settings due to their wired settings with alternative at-home options being less reliable and subject to user error. There are now a number of wearable sensors that can perform these functions in real time and almost continuously with the same or even greater degree of accuracy. Also, their connection to the internet sends the measured data into a cloud database. Some of these will be discussed in detail, along with their advantages and disadvantages, later on in this book. More importantly, we will discuss how they can be used to improve human health and performance on a daily basis in different environments.

Neurological Health

Neurological health involves the brain, the spinal cord, and 12 nerves that come from the brain. The nervous system can affect every part of the human body, so a thorough investigation of an individual's nervous system can indicate if there is neurological damage that can impede daily functioning. It can affect vision, hearing, sense of smell, sense of taste, and ability to speak as well as one's general mobility and cognitive function. These problems can be easily examined by a physician testing normal movements and reactions. Mental tests, motor function and balance, and sensory exams can be used to determine if neurological function is normal (Johns Hopkins Medicine, 2019).

If there is a greater issue with neurological health that goes beyond basic testing, health can be measured by some biological tests, the most notable biological test being the electroencephalogram (EEG) which monitors electrical activity in the brain. It can detect abnormalities because the normal activity of the brain creates a discernable pattern due to unique activities being controlled by specific parts of the brain. Slower frequencies are recorded when humans are drowsy and tired, and higher frequencies dominate when humans are hyper-alert. This biological test can help measure normal neurological functioning within the human brain (Sowndhararajan & Kim, 2016).

Behavioral Issues and Health

Behavioral and mental health are often linked, so it is very common for behavioral and mental issues to occur simultaneously. There is, however, an important distinction between the two types of health. Mental health impacts a person's emotional, psychological, and social wellbeing as well as nearly every aspect of one's life. Behavioral health focuses on how lifestyle habits can influence both physical and mental health. Good behavioral health practices can be beneficial to an individual's mental health, but can also influence other aspects of people's lives and mortality rates.

Adherence to healthy lifestyle behaviors is directly associated with decreased mortality. Those with four or more healthy behaviors lower their mortality up to 66% (Loef & Walach, 2012). King et al. (2009) define a healthy lifestyle by regular physical activity, adequate intake of fruits and vegetables, maintaining a healthy weight, and not smoking. Healthy habits and their benefits are not limited to those who have practiced these habits their whole life. Switching to a healthy lifestyle later in life can reduce an individual's risk of cardiovascular disease by 35% in just four years (King et al., 2009). Adherence to these habits can be an important indiciation of future public health trends and economic costs.

While these healthy behaviors are evidence-based, only a small portion of adults follow this lifestyle. Health risk behaviors such as tobacco use, alcohol consumption, physical inactivity, unhealthy diet, risky sexual behavior, and lack of disease screening can negatively affect human health. These lifestyle behaviors are associated with the development of some diseases such as cancer, heart disease, stroke, and diabetes (Lopez et al., 2006). Human behaviors, therefore, can positively or negatively impact an individual's health, and choosing to adhere to a healthy lifestyle can decrease mortality. Monitoring and having access to one's own health data via mobile tracking devices may benefit an individual's behavioral and lifestyle choices. Parts 2 and 3 will delve further into this discussion.

Psychological Health

A person's emotional, behavioral, and social maturity are important indicators of measuring health. Psychological health is commonly perceived as difficult to measure because of its complexity and ability to impact every area of one's life. In addition, there is limited availability of biological tests to measure psychological health and cultural differences within the framework of "normal". For these reasons, defining what is considered normal psychological health is a challenging task.

Psychological health is typically measured by a rigorous assessment performed by clinicians, psychiatrists, or clinical psychologists. There are two international standards for diagnosing mental illness: The World Health Organization's International Classification of Diseases version 10 (ICD-10), and the American Psychological Association's Diagnostic Statistical Manual version 5 (DSM-V). Both systems focus on similar symptoms that can rate loneliness, self-esteem, and happiness to diagnose a variety of mental health disorders such as depression, anxiety, post-traumatic stress disorder (PTSD), schizophrenia, eating disorders, and bipolar disorder (King, 2018).

There are disconnects between the two systems, but both are helpful measurement tools for mental health. Characterizing what is normal psychological health and what is abnormal psychological health is important. Abnormal thoughts, emotions, and behaviors categorize irregular behavioral and psychological measures.

Kinesthesiological Health

Kinesthesiology is the study of the movement of muscles and joints and one's perception of those motions. Muscles primarily function to produce motion, maintain posture, move internal organs, contract the heart, and aid in digestion. Normal muscle tissue will allow movement, respond to a stimulus, and react to that stimulus. Muscle movement can either be voluntary and under conscious control or be involuntary and not under conscious control (Betts et al., 2014).

There are three types of muscle tissue: Skeletal, cardiac, and smooth. Skeletal muscle is attached to the bone and is responsible for controlling locomotion, facial reactions, posture, and voluntary movements of the body. Cardiac muscle contracts on its own without any external stimulation to pump blood throughout the body. Smooth muscle controls involuntary movement of internal organs. It is found in the walls of major organs and helps with the movement of food and respiration, and regulates blood flow of arteries (Betts et al., 2014).

Human Sense and Perception

Human sense and perception are closely related. Sensing the environment involves touch, taste, sight, sound, and smell, while perceiving the environment is the interpretation of these sensations. Perception is conscious and depends on sensation; essentially, perception makes sense of the world around us based on the five senses. Many factors can influence human sense, recognition, and perception. The built environment is one important factor which can directly influence these sensations and perceptions, which indicates its design has the potential to influence an individual's wellbeing.

Smell

An individual's sense of smell is a chemical sense that helps identify food, danger, partners, and predators in communication with the environment. Pleasurable smells can elicit satisfaction, but smell can also act as a warning system that can alert one to danger. The stimulation of olfactory nerves and subsequent perception of odor can alter cognition, mood, and social behavior because olfaction stimulates interactions in the central nervous system (Strous & Shoenfeld, 2006).

Physiological and psychological effects of smell influence human sense and perception by playing an important role in mood, stress, and working capacity. Different odors have different impacts on mood. Lavender, for example, is considered a relaxing odor, whereas neroli is considered a stimulating odor (Campenni et al., 2004). This can impact humans physiologically because relaxing odors can decrease heart rate and skin conductance, whereas stimulating odors reverse these effects under the same or equivalent conditions. Inhalation of different aromas can stimulate different areas of the brain leading to a physiological response dependent on the brain's interpretation. Certain smells can cause alterations in both the emotions and behavior of a person (Sowndhararajan & Kim, 2016).

Sight

Visual information such as the perception of shapes, movement, color, and depth is collected by the sense of sight. The mind receives these visual cues when one is awake and alert. Interpreting the surrounding environment, surveying a visual scene, recognizing an object, and deciding on a plan of action based on this information require complex cognitive visual pathways that are processed in the temporal and parietal lobes and contribute to human sight (Das et al., 2007). Human vision and the sense of sight allow individuals to connect with their environment through visual information and stimulation. It is a sensory experience that sends signals to the brain that converts the information into images. Sight also impacts the brain in other ways, and stimulation of the visual cortex can influence other human perceptions such as pain.

Patients experiencing pain usually manage their pain through pharmacological management. However, human sight is a strong sensation, and the perception of images around a patient can be effective for pain management. Therapeutic virtual reality can transport patients into lifelike, three-dimensional worlds that stimulate the visual cortex and engage other senses. It acts as a distraction to other stimuli that may be causing the patient pain from procedures such as intravenous line placements and dental interventions. Engaging people in a positive and aesthetically pleasing visual built environment, therefore, is imperative (Spiegel et al., 2019).

Sound

Vibrations cause sound waves that travel to the ear and are then processed by the brain as sound. Distinctive sounds can elicit different responses which is why particular sounds can define a space as a positive or negative setting for human activity. Controlling the sensation of sound is so important because the interpretation of pleasurable sounds can promote good health while generally annoying sounds can impede health by disrupting sleep and causing irritability (Andringa & Lanser, 2013).

Quiet and pleasant environments promote a freedom of mind, allowing an individual to be in tune with the environment. Noise that is perceived as unpleasant increases hormones related to stress such as epinephrine, norepinephrine, and cortisol in the body (Babisch, 2002), while increasing the need for individuals to be vigilant and aware of their environment (Andringa & Lanser, 2013). Very loud and unexpected noises like military jets, speedboats, gunshots, loud music, or other city appliances are perceived as a negative and strongly increases the need for quietness (Booi & van den Berg, 2012).

In environments such as hospitals and other healthcare spaces, unwanted sounds may affect both the patient and staff's ability to hear and be heard, which can cultivate a threatening environment that potentially increases fear and anxiety levels. Specific architectural design can reduce the quantity of stressful sounds; an effective overall acoustical design, therefore, is fundamental to an individual's built environment. Acoustical design involves the consideration of sound transmission and sound absorption techniques. Sound transmission includes walls and ceilings that reduce sound transmission between spaces, whereas sound absorption involves sound-absorbing materials and finishes on walls, floors, and ceilings for public spaces such as corridors, congregation areas, and private spaces such as offices and patient rooms (Szántová & Rychtáriková, 2015).

Touch

The human skin's primary function is to act as a protective barrier to the outside world. The somatosensory system processes information that is in direct contact with an individual to generate a sense of touch. Direct contact with an object can convey information about texture and shape, which is why the sense of touch profoundly impacts the way humans view the world.

There are a variety of sensations that can be interpreted into information such as temperature, pain, or pressure. The sense of touch also has a sense of aesthetics when feeling surfaces that are particularly rough versus feeling a smooth surface. Humans may prefer the touch of a smooth surface compared to the touch of a rough surface or vice versa. The sense of touch is also closely related to visual stimulation, which can create the illusion of both pressure and thermal sensations (Gottfried, 2011).

Mental

Physical and mental health are fundamentally associated. Positive or negative mental health can directly influence one's physical health. Mental health includes emotional, psychological, and social wellbeing and can be affected by biological factors, life experiences, exercise, diet, and a family history of mental health. Positive mental health is important for individuals to cope with everyday stresses in life.

Healing environments influence a patient's wellbeing, which is why their design is so important. The design of the built environment can help manage the mental health and psychological wellbeing of individuals. Poorly designed environments may be detrimental to people in their daily lives. They may, however, have an even more pronounced negative effect on vulnerable populations such as those in psychiatric facilities. For example, furniture can be rearranged in psychiatric facilities to promote social interaction and decrease isolated and passive behaviors (Evans, 2003).

Human Wellbeing Indicators

Measurable and observable human wellbeing indicators include respiratory rate, skin temperature, sweating, heart rate variability (HRV), thermal comfort, visual comfort, sleep schedules, and mental performance. Any abnormalities outside of the normal range of these factors can potentially be indicative of health problems. Knowing what is normal and abnormal for human wellbeing is important to ensure a healthy and productive life.

Respiratory Rate

Respiration rates are measured typically when a person is at rest by measuring how many breaths they are taking per minute. The normal adult respiration rate for adults at rest is 12–20 breaths per minute. This means that any number of breaths under 12 or over 25 while at rest is considered abnormal. A variety of factors can influence these abnormalities such as asthma, anxiety, lung disease, fever, or other medical conditions (University of Rochester Medical Center, 2019).

Skin Temperature

Skin temperature is managed by the hypothalamus, part of the brain, to regulate body temperature (i.e., internal temperature). Temperature sensors in the skin send thermal information to this particulate part of the brain, where diverse physiological responses (e.g., blood flow to the skin, sweat, and shivering) are managed. Skin temperature beyond certain thresholds (upper and lower limits) causes pain by triggering the pain receptors. Also, it has a high correlation with physical activities and ambient temperature. With support of such mechanisms, internal temperature should be managed properly; otherwise, serious health issues could arise (e.g., brain damage, cardiac arrhythmia, and death).

Sweat

Sweat glands cover the human body and can vary based on gender, age, genetic makeup, and athletic ability. There are a few reasons why increased sweat is considered normal. When an individual overheats, becomes nervous or anxious, or is exercising, sweating more than normal is an effective tool for thermoregulation. This is considered normal and healthy because all thermoregulation mechanisms are designed to return one's body to homeostasis or equilibrium, which is essential for a human cells' health.

Excessive sweating due to abnormalities of the human body can be linked to fever, stress, obesity, menopause, heart attack, or other medical problems. Heavy sweating that accompanies chills, lightheadedness, chest pain, nausea, or fever is indicative of needing to contact a doctor. People with excessive sweating should seek a doctor when sweating disrupts routine, causes emotional distress, or occurs at night for no reason (Mayo Clinic, 2018).

Heart Rate Variability

A healthy pulse range for adults is 60–100 beats per minute. There are both healthy irregularities and unhealthy irregularities when measuring heart rate. Heart rate is not constant and can vary in time and strength. This variation is controlled by the autonomic nervous system which acts unconsciously to regulate different bodily functions. HRV should be checked because it can be used to identify imbalances that can be caused by stress, poor sleep, lack of exercise, and an unhealthy diet. High HRV can be indicative of greater cardiovascular fitness and resilience to stress. The most conventional and accurate way to check HRV has been using an electrocardiogram (ECG) which measures the electrical activity of the heart rate. It is beneficial to understand what is normal to understand how to respond to the stresses of life in increasingly beneficial ways (Campos, 2017). It is now, however, quite common to use a number of noninvasive sensors on the human body (usually wrist- or chest-worn) to measure heart rate accurately and in real time. Although they have been widely used to measure human performance in military personnel and athletes, they are now being increasingly used to measure productivity in office workers, and to monitor and predict health and performance in special populations such as older adults or even regular people who are concerned about their everyday health. We will discuss some of these devices further in this book.

Thermal Comfort

The American Society of Heating, Refrigerating and Air-Conditioning Engineers (ASHRAE) defines thermal comfort as "condition of mind that expresses satisfaction with the thermal environment and is assessed by subjective evaluation" (ASHRAE Standard 55, 2017). This indicator is one of the primary purposes of heating, ventilation, and air-conditioning (HVAC) in a building. As defined, it involves a variety of environmental and human factors and often leaves up to individuals' preferences; therefore, it is challenging to be generalized. Conventionally, the perception of being thermally neutral was considered desirable (Fanger, 1970), but diversity in preferred environmental conditions has been demonstrated by literature (Humphreys & Hancock, 2007). Also, literature established that there is a certain range of temperature, where people perform better.

Visual Comfort

Visual comfort can be measured quantitatively and qualitatively. When it comes to a quantitative evaluation, illuminance (i.e., the amount of light falling onto a given surface area) is a commonly used metric, although luminance (i.e., the amount of light leaving a surface) represents the actual light level that people see. A certain level of light required for visual comfort and glare for example, disturbs observers due to the excessive contrast or an inappropriate distribution of light sources. A qualitative measure could include three components: content, access, and clarity (Ko et al., 2021), and it can associate with physiology, psychology (e.g., mood), and beyond.

Sleep

On average, human adults should be receiving seven or more hours of sleep each night. If an individual receives less than seven hours of sleep, it has been found to constitute a short sleep duration. Sleep disorders and dysfunction are prevalent in the United States and vary based on age, sex, and race. There are behavioral and chronic health risks associated with short sleep duration. Adults who sleep for short periods of time are more likely to report physical inactivity, smoking habits, and obesity and have an increased risk of chronic health conditions (Centers for Disease Control and Prevention, 2010).

Sleep disorders can be associated with the built environment due to varying types and levels of light exposures and excessive noise, traffic, or air pollution (Johnson et al., 2018). Sleep disorders can directly impact an individual's health because it can decrease productivity, influence the operation of motor vehicles, and contribute to an increased risk of chronic health conditions.

Mental Performance

Mental performance is also an inherent part of physical performance and health. Individuals that are in a state of normal mental health have basic cognitive social skills, can mediate their emotions concerning others, and can efficiently cope with unaccepted and adverse life events. Mental health disruptions can cause alterations in behavior, mood, and thinking, which are associated with impaired functioning. Unique, individual factors can affect the mental health of each person in specific ways. Every person has experiences, societal structures, and cultural values that can contribute to mental health differently based on certain risk factors that increase the risk of mental health issues. The presence of abnormal mental performance can be a result of a variety of mental health issues such as anxiety, depression, and PTSD (Galderisi et al., 2015).

A thorough review of existing research in the field of health and the built environment resulted in finding different human health measures, human sense and perception, and wellbeing indicators in different settings. Defining normal health in the context of this chapter was important before analyzing how human senses, perceptions, experiences, and health outcomes can be impacted by the built environment. Research on new technologies to measure health and wellbeing outcomes in built environments needs to be interdisciplinary, requiring collaboration across the fields of design, planning, medicine, public health, environmental, social and behavioral sciences, data analytics, and computer sciences. There is increasing evidence showing how built environments impact our health, and therefore, considering how evidence-based design can make a significant difference to our lives is urgently required.

References

American Society of Heating, Refrigerating and Air-Conditioning Engineers (ASHRAE). (2017). Thermal Environmental Conditions for Human Occupancy. ASHRAE Standard 55.

Andringa, T., & Lanser, J. (2013). How pleasant sounds promote and annoying sounds impede health: A cognitive approach. *International Journal of Environmental Research and Public Health*, *10*(4), 1439–1461.

Babisch, W. (2002). The noise/stress concept, risk assessment and research needs. *Noise and Health*, *4*(16), 1.

Betts, J. G., Desaix, P., Johnson, E., Johnson, J. E., Koral, O., Kruse, D., ... & Young, K. A. (2013). Anatomy & physiology. (2013). *Open Stax College*, *1*(1), 1–1.

Booi, H., & van den Berg, F. (2012). Quiet areas and the need for quietness in Amsterdam. *International Journal of Environmental Research and Public Health*, *9*(4), 1030–1050.

Campenni, C. E., Crawley, E. J., & Meier, M. E. (2004). Role of suggestion in odor-induced mood change. *Psychological Reports*, *94*(3 Pt 2), 1127–1136. https://doi.org/10.2466/pr0.94.3c.1127-1136

Campos, M. (2017, November 22). Heart rate variability: A new way to track wellbeing. Retrieved from https://www.health.harvard.edu/blog/heart-rate-variability-new-way-track-well-2017112212789

Centers for Disease Control and Prevention. (2010, February). Sleep and sleep disorders. Retrieved from https://www.cdc.gov/sleep/data_statistics.html

Das, M., Bennett, D. M., & Dutton, G. N. (2007). Visual attention as an important visual function: An outline of manifestations, diagnosis and management of impaired visual attention. *British Journal of Ophthalmology*, *91*(11), 1556–1560.

Evans, G. W. (2003). The built environment and mental health. *Journal of Urban Health*, *80*(4), 536–555.

Fanger, P. O. (1970). *Thermal comfort: Analysis and applications in environmental engineering*. Copenhagen: Danish Technical Press.

Galderisi, S., Heinz, A., Kastrup, M., Beezhold, J., & Sartorius, N. (2015). Toward a new definition of mental health. *World Psychiatry*, *14*(2), 231–233.

Gottfried, J. A. (2011). *Neurobiology of sensation and reward*. CRC Press, New York.

Humphreys, M. A., & Hancock, M. (2007). Do people like to feel 'neutral'?: Exploring the variation of the desired thermal sensation on the ASHRAE scale. *Energy and Buildings*, *39*(7), 867–874.

Johns Hopkins Medicine. (2019). Neurological exam. Retrieved from https://www.hopkinsmedicine.org/health/conditions-and-diseases/neurological-exam

Johnson, D. A., Hirsch, J. A., Moore, K. A., Redline, S., & Diez Roux, A. V. (2018). Associations between the built environment and objective measures of sleep: The multi-ethnic study of Atherosclerosis. *American Journal of Epidemiology*, *187*(5), 941–950.

King, D. E., Mainous III, A. G., Carnemolla, M., & Everett, C. J. (2009). Adherence to healthy lifestyle habits in US adults, 1988–2006. *The American Journal of Medicine*, *122*(6), 528–534.

King, J. (2018, February). Measuring mental health outcomes in built environment research. Retrieved from https://www.urbandesignmentalhealth.com/how-to-measure-mental-health.html

Ko, W. H., Kent, M. G., Schiavon, S., Levitt, B., & Betti, G. (2021). A window view quality assessment framework. *LEUKOS, The Journal of the Illuminating Engineering Society, 18*(3), 268–293.

Loef, M., & Walach, H. (2012). The combined effects of healthy lifestyle behaviors on all cause mortality: A systematic review and meta-analysis. *Preventive Medicine, 55*(3), 163–170.

Lopez, A. D., Mathers, C. D., Ezzati, M., Jamison, D. T., & Murray, C. J. (2006). Global and regional burden of disease and risk factors, 2001: Systematic analysis of population health data. *The Lancet, 367*(9524), 1747–1757.

Mayo Clinic. (2018, June 21). Excessive sweating when to see a doctor. Retrieved from https://www.mayoclinic.org/symptoms/excessive-sweating/basics/when-to-see-doctor/sym-20050780.

Sowndhararajan, K., & Kim, S. (2016). Influence of fragrances on human psychophysiological activity: With special reference to human electroencephalographic response. *Scientiapharmaceutica, 84*(4), 724–751.

Spiegel, B., Fuller, G., Lopez, M., Dupuy, T., Noah, B., Howard, A., ... & Dailey, F. (2019). Virtual reality for management of pain in hospitalized patients: A randomized comparative effectiveness trial. *PloS One, 14*(8), e0219115.

Strous, R. D., & Shoenfeld, Y. (2006). To smell the immune system: Olfaction, autoimmunity and brain involvement. *Autoimmunity Reviews, 6*(1), 54–60.

Szántová, G., & Rychtáriková, M. (2015). The importance of audio-visual aspects in the architectural design of psychiatric clinics. *Energy Procedia, 78*, 1251–1256.

University of Rochester Medical Center. (2019). Vital signs (Body Temperature, Pulse Rate, Respiration Rate, Blood Pressure). Retrieved from https://www.urmc.rochester.edu/encyclopedia/content.aspx?ContentTypeID=85&ContentID=P00866

2 Environmental Measures

Introduction

This chapter provides a comprehensive overview of environmental fundamentals necessary to inform health, wellbeing, and performance (Figure 2.1). The range of environmental factors influencing built environment conditions are discussed, including air quality, light, acoustic, thermal, and spatio-material measures. Each of these variables has a profound influence on the human experience and thus human health and wellbeing. In some cases, these environmental variables present stressors to humans, while, in other cases, the environment can aid and support human healing and wellbeing. The first section, "Environment Types," discusses a few different built environment typologies we typically encounter in our lives and how they influence human health. The second section, "Environmental Measures," delves into different scientific ways of characterizing different variables that affect comfort, health, and productivity in these environments.

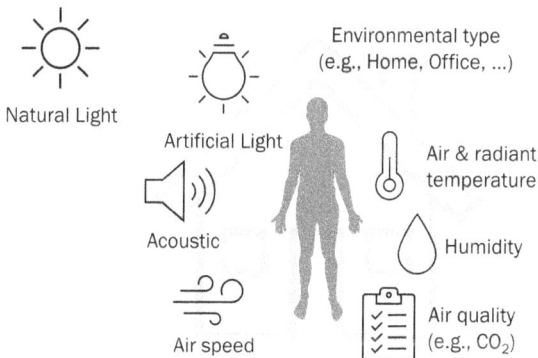

Figure 2.1 Composite Diagram: Interscalar Environmental Variables Influencing Human Health in and around Buildings.

DOI: 10.4324/9780367814748-4

Environment Types

Outdoor, Urban Environments

An urban area typically has a high population density and is greatly affected by the built environment which is composed of urban design, land use, and the transportation systems of a city, all of which incorporate human activity. Urban design refers to the arrangement and appearance of physical elements combined with the overall design of the city. Land use typically includes the location, distribution, and different categories of activities such as residential, commercial, office, and industrial. The transportation system is influenced by the physical infrastructure of roads, sidewalks, bike paths, bridges, and more (Handy et al., 2002).

The field of public health and urban planning shares a common goal of improving human health and wellbeing by focusing on increasing public safety and accessibility. The use of urban planning to improve overall public health can be seen through a variety of design elements. For example, design elements of the transportation system of an area have the potential to improve air quality, increase the amount of physical activity, and prevent injuries from occurring (Kochtitzky et al., 2006). Urban planning to promote the amount of physical activity of an area can occur through street connectivity and overall design elements. Promoting physical activity through the design of the built environment will help create active and healthier communities (Handy et al., 2002). Urban design that decreases the amount of physical activity of a community increases the health risks associated with obesity and related conditions such as diabetes, and poor mental and cardiovascular health (World Health Organization, 2018).

Frank and Engelke (2001) provide support for the public health benefits associated with urban planning such as improvements in regional mobility, traffic congestion, and air quality. If human health and activity is emphasized, urban planning can be used to encourage two forms of moderate physical activity: walking and biking. Transportation systems in urban environments determine the physical pathways. For example, bikeways, railways, and sidewalks are all related to whether an individual will obtain increased physical activity. A grid pattern generally reduces the amount of walking and biking an individual must do so it created high connectivity and likelihood someone will bike rather than drive (Frank & Engelke, 2001).

The planning of land use in cities can also determine how local neighborhoods and communities influence health and wellbeing. A study by Kyttä et al. (2012) found that residential density in a child-friendly urban setting was associated with active travel, active behavioral patterns, and therefore health benefits. Environmental child-friendliness includes characteristics that increase both the diversity in environmental resources and the access to play and exploration. Urban planning and characteristics in the environment can promote activity and mobility within children. Children and parents who perceive an environment to be unsafe will decrease their mobility in that environment and subsequent behavior that encourages them to be active. Policies should strive to encourage the use of public spaces for physical activity because the urban environment can increase active behavioral patterns (Kyttä et al., 2012).

Most of the world's population spends a majority of their time indoors so the standards that dictate the design and construction of buildings affect health, safety, and security of those who reside in them. Poor urban planning can cause preventable injuries, death, and destruction of buildings in countries that are experiencing rapid urbanization because these buildings can be riddled with building code violations. Poor-quality design can be caused by out-of-date or lack of comprehensive building codes and standards, the failure to obtain necessary approvals, and the use of poor-quality materials. Complying to building codes can prevent disease, injury, and death, and promote safety. Building collapses and fires due to poor urban planning can cause preventable injuries, death, and destruction of buildings (Chauvin et al., 2016).

A study by Galea et al. (2005) analyzed the association between an urban neighborhood, and the likelihood of depression. This study conducted a random telephone survey on the residents of the New York City metropolitan area. The study found that people living in neighborhoods that were characterized as poorer were more likely to report both past six-month depression and lifetime depression. The researchers explained this by relating the psychosocial stress found in these poorer urban neighborhoods to substantial stressors that can be directly tied to deteriorating built environments. In addition, these residents are exposed to a grater rate of noise, violence, and trauma, which can also be associated with poor mental health. (Galea et al., 2005). Overall, this study showed that characteristics of the built environment are associated with the likelihood of depression. This means that urban planners and public health professionals should work together to identify potential ideas that would improve the health and wellbeing of its residents through urban planning.

Indoor Environments

According to the National Research Council (1981), approximately 90% of an average person's day is spent in enclosed areas where the concentration of pollutants is relatively higher than outside. The indoors typically refer to environments in homes, cars, schools, workplaces, public buildings, and other spaces where the public has access such as stores or restaurants. Enhancing indoor environmental quality should be a key priority in the design, operation, or renovation of a building to provide a foundation for healthier lives. Effective design and construction of indoor spaces supports health and wellbeing with safe, comfortable, and pollution-free spaces (Urban Land Institute, McCormick et al., 2013).

There are a variety of factors that impact the quality of indoor air, including the ventilation system, lighting and heating/cooling devices, types of furnishings, tobacco smoking by occupants, pesticides, cooking, home appliances, or the infiltration of outside air. Additionally, humans are exposed to a variety of indoor pollutants such as radon, formaldehyde, asbestos, and moisture and mold (National Research Council, 1981). Poor indoor air quality is associated with allergies, weakened immune systems, irritation, and illness, especially when people are exposed to high concentrations of these toxins. It can negatively impact both cardiovascular and respiratory health. These environments are predominately created mostly by a combination of occupants' activities and the intrusion of outdoor pollutants (World Health Organization, 2018).

Building construction materials may have behavioral toxins such as heavy metals, pesticides, and solvents that have neurological and cognitive impacts that can impact psychological wellbeing. Lead impedes attention and frustration tolerance in children, which can result in irritability and aggression. Hazardous materials such as mercury and organic solvents have been linked to anxiety, depression, and concentration difficulties. Threats to health based on indoor air pollution can cause psychological distress and heightened family conflicts (Evans, 2003). Eliminating and decreasing indoor air pollutants, therefore, is essential for increasing indoor air quality and maintaining the physical and mental health of the residents

Workplace

Workplace culture has undergone many transformations in the last three decades. Technological developments and emphasis on collaboration have led to work settings where individuals work more dynamically. Technical innovations and economic pressures have created a need for work settings to be agile, adapt to changing market conditions, and optimal for productivity and performance (Harris, 2015). Productivity, therefore, is a major concern in workplaces today. It affects business profit margins, return on investment (ROI), and ultimately the value of the company.

As investors and business look at ways to meet these demands, they are beginning to consider workplaces that are flexible and adaptable to enable workers to customize their office experience (Harris, 2015). Customization, however, needs to include not only better user controls of the environment but also design elements that respond to user needs for reducing stress which is directly related to improving health, productivity, and performance (Lamb & Kwok, 2015).

Stress in our everyday lives comes from several different situations which may be from factors that are social (e.g., work demands from an employer), physical (e.g., long hours or manual labor), or biological and chemical (e.g., headache, nausea, or fatigue due to emissions from carpet, paint, or other interior materials and finishes). Stress, therefore, may be a psychological or physiological response to a stimulus or a "stressor" in an individual's surrounding environment (Donald & Siu, 2001).

Stress may also be of the internal or external variety (Marion, 2003). Internal stressors include violence, conflict, or disorganization, while external stressors include physical environmental variables such as noise, temperature, humidity, light, and over- or under-stimulation. Stress can build over time and lead to physical or mental illness (Kopec, 2006). Designers can play an active role in minimizing stress at the workplace by determining how these environmental variables are accounted for during the pre-design, design, and construction phases, and how they can be controlled or operated.

Building design has a strong connection to workers' wellbeing and productivity as revealed by a study funded by the US Department of Energy (Heerwagen, 1998). It concluded that a building could be successful only if it was successful in satisfying its occupants. Heerwagen conceptualized that ability, motivation, and opportunity were the three dimensions of human performance, which in turn were affected by building design. "Ability," as defined by Heerwagen, was whether a person could perform a task; "motivation" was whether that person wanted to do it; and "opportunity" was whether there were accessible means to accomplish that task. Her study concluded that buildings could positively affect all three dimensions. As frustrating as employee absenteeism may be for office managers, they need to step back and consider whether the major reason for this behavior is a lack of motivation to come in every day.

Designers need to work closely with health-care professionals to shape building design and operation policy, standards, and guidelines to prevent diseases from transferring and to protect workers. This includes architects, planners, and engineers using US national guidelines such as the American Society of Heating, Refrigerating and Air-Conditioning Engineers (ASHRAE), and the Occupational Safety and Health Administration (OSHA). Some states such as California have specific guidelines and standards (O'Hara et al., 2018). Setting standards, best practices, and policies, however, requires a data-driven approach to collect objective measurements of living and working environments, and individual health.

Home

A variety of complex factors affect an individual's health at home. Inadequate and substandard housing is a major public health issue. According to the housing and health guidelines of the World Health Organization (WHO), safe housing conditions support a state of complete physical, social, and mental wellbeing by providing accessibility, comfortable temperatures, and safety from injuries. Healthy housing conditions can pertain to the physical structure, the community, and the immediate housing environment. The physical structure can impact human health by being structurally sound, promoting appropriate temperatures, and providing protection from unsanitary conditions, injury hazards, and pollutants. The local community can encourage healthy social interactions to support physical, social, and mental wellbeing. Finally, the immediate housing environment can provide access to public transportation options and different services, and protect an individual from waste or natural disaster (World Health Organization, 2018). Proper attention to these issues can create a healthy housing environment.

Epidemiological findings suggest that human health is strongly associated with adequate shelter, which is why housing quality can have a profound effect on health (Bonnefoy, 2007). Living in adequate shelter means having a place that protects privacy and provides elements that support both physical and psychological wellbeing. The quality and adequacy of one's housing varies based on cultural, social, and environmental contexts as well as age and gender-specific factors (Bonnefoy, 2007). This is what makes the home such a complex construct and why there are a variety of factors that can impact the quality of life of a resident. One of the primary goals of housing is to act as a buffer and provide protection from outside aggression. When housing fails at providing sufficient protection, it allows its inhabitants to feel intruded upon. Bonnefoy (2007) concluded that this leads to feelings that affect mental health such as anxiety, depression, insomnia, and social dysfunction. Subjective satisfaction in the home is important because it contributes to psychosocial wellbeing and overall mental health. The home has the potential to be an environment that people attach their identity to and find refuge from outside stressors (Bonnefoy, 2007). This is heavily impacted by both the characteristics of the home and overall stability of an individual's housing situation.

An increasing body of evidence directly links housing quality to increased morbidity from infectious diseases, chronic illnesses, injuries, poor nutrition, and mental disorders (Krieger & Higgins, 2002). Substandard housing has features that impair the health of a person due to inadequate water quality, air quality, neighborhood noise, and tobacco smoke. These poor housing features can increase exposure to health risks. Poor construction or maintenance can increase the risk of injury, lack of accessibility potentially increases feelings of stress and isolation, and crowded housing can increase exposure to infectious disease (World Health Organization, 2018). Inadequate housing, therefore, can influence every aspect of an individual's life and overall health.

Physical, social, and mental health are inherently linked. When one form of health is adversely affected, it leads to the disruption of other forms of health. Physical health describes the visible condition and health of one's body, and it is critical to wellbeing. Residential environments can impact physical health in a variety of ways and therefore have an impact on mental health as well. Physical and tangible features of an individual's home such as excessive indoor temperature are linked with irritability and social intolerance. Furthermore, damp, moldy, and cold indoor conditions are associated with an increased risk of anxiety and depression (Krieger & Higgins, 2002).

Virtual

Jerdan et al. (2018) define virtual reality (VR) as a technological medium that displays a three-dimensional and computer-generated environment that is viewed through a head-mounted display. An immersive VR system allows users to interact within the three-dimensional, computer-generated world and has implications on human health and wellbeing. It is rapidly making progress in the health-care industry as it becomes increasingly affordable and accessible to individuals. The emerging research in VR shows that it is proving to be an effective tool for both physical and mental aspects of human health (Jerdan et al., 2018).

There are a few key figures that are important when discussing the beginnings of VR. The term "VR" was originally coined by Jaron Lanier in 1987, but the development of VR first arose when cinematographer Morton Heilig built the Sensorama to stimulate the senses of the audience during films. The Sensorama, though not interactive, consisted of a stereoscopic color display, fans, a sound system, and odor emitters. It was not until the 1990s that VR was first used in medical teaching to assist with colonoscopy and upper gastrointestinal tract endoscopy simulations. It is currently being used in the field of health care in two different ways: as a simulation tool primarily used by physicians and surgeons, and as an interaction tool primarily used in behavioral health medicine. There are a wide variety of VR techniques that are beneficial to health care such as diagnosis, treatment, rehabilitation, counseling, and even designing hospitals (Srivastava et al., 2014).

VR is immersive and interactive, and can be beneficial because it changes the way humans interact with their immediate environment. Humans perceive their environment using the five senses: vision, hearing, touch, taste, and smell. VR delivers sensory information through a head-mounted display allowing for complete immersion into the computer-generated environment (Maples-Keller et al., 2017). VR has the potential to be an effective and valuable tool when designing health-care facilities because it can strengthen the communication between design teams and future building users and allow designers to experience the space during any phase of the project, thereby accelerating decision-making and saving time, money, and resources. Engaging clients and building designers can strengthen the field of VR in relation to built environments and health, and yield positive results (McAllister, 2014).

Rizzo (2003) argued that VR can also have direct positive effects on human health and wellbeing by immersing physical therapy patients in interactive environments. VR offers the unique opportunity to bring the complex physical world into a controlled laboratory setting. Through this, the ability to create a synthetic and computer-generated environment offers several positive effects for the rehabilitation of patients. Physical therapy can feel repetitive and tedious to recovering patients, but technological advances seen in VR can be interesting and compelling. The potential to instantly be notified of recovery milestones such as buttoning a shirt for the first time after a stroke, users playing games that enhance motivation, and training in a variety of simulated environments are a few ways that VR can ultimately aid in physical therapy and motor rehabilitation. Providing safe, interactive, and stimulating training environments that can also be duplicated and distributed at a low cost are a few benefits of VR in the health field (Rizzo, 2003).

Health-Care Environments

Environments to improve health and treat illnesses and disease may at times, ironically, be very stressful spaces to visit, stay for short or longer periods of time, or work on a daily basis. Patients experience a considerable amount of stress due to medical procedures that are painful; there can be loss of independence and autonomy, loss of control over their environments, or temporary loss of social relationships. While many of these stressors are related to health-care organization and management culture, a considerable amount are due to poorly designed environments. These include spaces that are noisy, have wayfinding difficulties, lack views to the outside, result in a loss of privacy, or are not conducive to family visits (Ulrich et al., 2006).

Stress in health-care environments has been found to influence the wellbeing of nurses and other staff as well. Besides increasing work demands, rotating shifts, and patient death, workspaces that are noisy, layouts that increase fatigue, and environments that lack adequate employee break and rest areas have also been found to negatively impact health-care employees (Ulrich et al., 2006).

A study by C. Douglas (2003) and M. Douglas (2003) analyzed four clinical areas in health-care environments, namely, surgery, medicine, maternity, and care of the elderly, and found similarities in their priorities and areas of concern. They found the most important themes in these four clinical areas to be a sense of privacy and personal space, a welcoming atmosphere, accessibly and comfortability of the physical design, access to outdoor areas such as fresh air and communal gardens, recreational facilities, and effective communication between the staff, patients, and relatives. The role of built environments in health care has a major effect on all these themes, as suggested by this study. Prioritizing these concerns can help make the hospital a supportive built environment for its residents.

Assessing common themes and similarities across all at-risk groups of the human population is, therefore, important to the architecture and overall built environment of hospitals. Care of the elderly is an extremely important area to address since the population of older adults in the world (aged 65+) is rapidly increasing. Detailed criteria for a senior-friendly hospital need to be developed because a large percentage of the hospital population is used by the elderly, and the prevalence of frailty and morbidity in older persons is higher (Rashmi et al., 2016). Maintaining a safe and age-friendly environment in the hospital is dependent upon the design of the built environments, its infrastructure, and specialized training and experience in geriatrics among staff.

Environmental Measures

Our environment consists of all aspects and contents of material, phenomena, and space that surrounds us at any given time. An environment can be physical or virtual or both simultaneously, but the primary focus of this section addresses physical built environment variables. These variables consist of air, light, sound, heat, and materials. Each variable, whether indoors or outdoors, is influenced by spatial conditions. It is important to have a basic understanding of the environmental fundamentals that influence our human experiences. These environmental conditions comprise the matrix for health and wellbeing responsiveness in designed indoor and outdoor spaces.

Differentiating between human comfort, human health, and human productivity or performance is significant for particular environmental measures. Human comfort is that which provides a satisfied state of mind based on environmental experience. For comfort, there is a direct link between the physiological and psychological experiences. Human health measures are strictly dependent on variables that impact our biological and physiological conditions. The research findings related to human health constitute higher precision and often narrower ranges of environmental values compared to what might be acceptable for comfort. Human performance and productivity measure the output of human activity as impacted by environmental conditions. In these scenarios, there are currently fewer conclusive research studies, and much of the data is directly tied to human comfort measures. However, methods and techniques for acquiring research data on human productivity and performance are addressed in Section "Outdoor, Urban Environments". In all scenarios, there are obvious challenges and limitations to achieve conclusive findings due to the nature of human subject research and isolation of complex variables. This section specifically addresses the environmental variables independent from human complexities.

Air Quality

Oxygen is necessary for human existence and is ascertained through our urban and indoor air. The quality of air in the environment is dependent upon emissions, materials, and microbiological factors. Research indicates that the quality of air chemistry and the amount of fresh air exchanges in buildings can have a significant impact on human wellbeing and performance (Fang et al., 2004). Outdoor urban environments have air quality challenges as a result of high emissions from vehicles that increase the carbon dioxide and nitrogen oxide levels, both of which are problematic to human wellbeing (Kemp et al., 2003). Indoor environments have air quality challenges resulting from both the materials and the modes of ventilation. Materials in buildings may off-gas volatile organic compounds (VOCs) and other chemicals that are problematic to human health. Ventilation in buildings often requires filtration methods that require ongoing maintenance and cleaning. Furthermore, the rate of air exchange between the outdoor and indoor environments can affect the quality of the indoor air. Higher rates of air exchange provide more continuous fresh air volume to building occupants, however, this will typically require an increase in energy consumption to run fans and ventilation equipment. The quality of air that we breath is also comprised of moisture, which influences the humidity levels. For human comfort, the relative humidity range should fall between 20% and 80%. However, for optimal human health, it is recommended that the relative humidity percentage be as close to 40% as possible (Taylor & Hugentobler, 2016).

Air quality is also comprised of biological entities that define our microbiome in the urban and indoor environments. This field of research is expanding as we learn that there are hundreds of thousands of microbiological entities that we are not yet aware and that are newly emerging through evolutionary processes in conjunction with new sensing techniques. It is important to acknowledge that there is a distinction to be made between helpful and harmful biological factors. Harmful entities include pathogens as well as airborne mold spores and allergens (Wolkoff, 2018). In prior studies on microbiomes, the research shows that fresh outdoor air contains healthier constituents than indoor air filtered through mechanical ventilation (Leung, 2015). Indoor air that is transferred through a means of natural ventilation is generally shown to be comprised of healthier microbiological constituents than mechanically ventilated air.

Numerous research studies have been conducted for indoor air quality and human health impacts. This established field of research informed characterizations of sick building syndrome in the 1980s and has since been leveraged to required new standards and expectations of building material compositions from the manufacturing industries. The research has also informed updated building codes for ventilation standards. As we continue to learn more about the composition and quality of our air, as well as the techniques to manage air exchange and ventilation, we can expect to move towards healthier built environments that provide not just clean air but also healthy air. The aromatics of air influences human experience and perception and can provide psychological benefits that impact the human physiology over time. The future air in our built environments may be monitored more closely with real-time sensing and response, and may provide an infusion of healthy probiotics and aromatics for medicinal effect.

Light

Light is comprised of electromagnetic energy provided by the sun or an electric lighting source. The visible spectrum falls between 380 nm and 740 nm wavelengths and provides an energy level that is perceptible to the human eye. The wavelength range begins at violet at the short wavelength end and moves through indigo, blue, green, yellow, orange, and red at the long wavelength end of the spectrum. The color of light is perceived because of its energy-band intensity that enters the iris of the eye and hits the retina to affect rods and cones, which then transmit signals to the human brain. Visual perception in the built environment requires a source of light and is affected by the color and intensity of light as well as the material colors, textures, and geometries. Light interacts with materials in the built environment through basic radiation mechanisms: reflectance, transmittance, absorptance, and emittance.

Access and exposure to light is fundamental for biological functions. Natural daylight provides significant benefits to humans in relationship to the signals that the brain receives that connect to the circadian rhythm and synchronize the wake and sleep cycles of human physiology. In certain geographic locations, the diurnal symmetry of daylight and night is skewed and may greatly limit the access to light at certain times of year. Societies in northern climate locations have greater rates of seasonal affective disorder (SAD) due to the limited exposure to sunlight during winter seasons (Melrose, 2015). Concurrently, some aspects of sunlight can be harmful to human health, such as overexposure to ultraviolet (UV) rays. When cells in the human body are exposed to UV, there is a chance for mutation of the cell structure, which can result in the development of cancers.

Architects, engineers, and building scientists have a broad and deep body of research around light and its interactions in buildings and with building occupants. Zoning codes in cities evolved in part to ensure direct access to daylight on building interiors by establishing solar envelope relationships (Saratsis et al., 2016). Glazing systems have received a lot of advancement and attention in order to allow for building enclosures that will maximize the amount of available daylight while simultaneously limiting the transmission of UV and heat gain. Both the quantitative and qualitative aspects of light are considered fundamental for building occupancy functions, and the discipline has evolved numerous modes for measuring, analyzing, and designing with light.

Acoustic

The acoustic environment influences human hearing and cognitive responsiveness (Lee & Jeon, 2013). Sound propagates through molecules in the air and materials. The concentric propagation patterns of sound, based on the fourth power law, influence the intensity of the pressures of phonon vibrations. Higher intensity occurs directly adjacent of the source of sound, with decreasing phonon vibration and pressure moving away from the source. Sound waves consist of a frequency and tone, or decibel range. The frequency is equivalent to the wavelength in the electromagnetic spectrum, with sound waves occurring at a much slower speed or rate in comparison with light and radiation.

The space and composition of materials informs the propagation of sound, including its behaviors and interactions with the environment. Sound may be absorbed, transmitted, reflected, and emitted from materials and sources just in the same way that light and radiation have these behaviors. The difference is in the directionality of energy transfer. Since sound travels in a lattice vibration path through molecules (and cannot move through a vacuum in the way that radiation or light can), it transmits along a three-dimensional conical path rather than a vector-based trajectory.

Absorption of sound into materials depends upon the amount of porosity in a material: the higher the porosity, the greater the ability to absorb sound (Arenas & Crocker, 2010). The reflection of sound off of surfaces is dependent primarily on the geometry and surface texture of the materials. Materials that are shaped in convex forms will redirect reflected sound in a focused way, while concave forms will spread sound outward across a greater area. Sound can be transmitted around materials and geometries based on the propagation path.

The qualities of sound that are experienced by human perception include tone, volume, and frequency. The human ear drum is a surface that receives the pressure of a sound wave and transmits that signal through the ear canal to the neuro-receptors in the brain for interpretation. Hearing loss and disabilities may affect the quality of sound experienced by a person, and thus their quality of wellbeing (Tambs, 2004). Noise in the built environment can become distracting to human concentration and focus, and in some cases, damaging to human hearing. Standards for acceptable human exposures to acoustic decibel levels are established for the built environment and also influence aspects of building design. Building enclosure systems can be designed to improve the acoustic separation between potentially noisy outdoor environments and the indoor occupied spaces. Acoustic partition systems for walls and floors for multi-occupancy buildings are devised to reduce sound transmission between different habitable spaces. Vibration from mechanical equipment in buildings can cause noise disturbances by transfer through building structures, which can be alleviated by the integration of noise dampening and sound isolation pads and materials.

Thermal

The thermal environment is often characterized by the temperature of the air, often measured via a dry-bulb temperature (DBT) sensor by, for example, thermostats. However, the human experience of perception of thermal conditions may be more greatly affected by radiant surfaces and materials. Mean radiant temperature (MRT) is the sum of exposures to emittance and radiation from surrounding materials and sources and largely influences human thermal comfort. Conduction between the human body and contact with materials in the building, or furniture, can also have a great impact on the experience of the thermal environment. Humidity levels also influence thermal conditions, as moisture in the air serves as a heat sink for the sensible heat and can enable a reduction of DBT to provide a cooling effect to humans. Air movement can also influence the human experience of thermal conditions. When air is moving across the surface of the skin, it will induce transpiration and provide a cooling effect via mostly convection. When air moves too quickly across surfaces of the human body, such as high-speed winds, the body can experience discomfort of the thermal environment. These four environmental factors are often taken into consideration when it comes to thermal environments.

While the sun is the global resource for providing temperature balance to our earth and heat and energy and light to our built and natural environments, we have evolved to depend on many other sources of energy to provide thermal conditioning. The values of thermal comfort for humans are based on research from the 1950s, especially the renowned predicted mean vote model (Fanger, 1967) and adaptive model (de Dear & Brager, 1998), whereas the present establishes data through mixed methods (Ličina et al., 2018). Qualitative surveys determine the perception, and state of mind, of human's experience of the thermal environment. Physiological measures determine the quantitative limits of thermal comfort and human health, and physical activities often play a significant role in thermal comfort. The human body must maintain a stable core temperature to maintain its health and functioning. The thermal environment plays a significant role in this aspect of human wellbeing.

Recent studies shed light on the possibility of modeling individual preferences in thermal comfort using participatory sensing (Jazizadeh et al., 2014) and/or wearable physiological sensors (Jung & Jazizadeh, 2018). Online survey platforms and the increase in connected devices have streamlined perception-related data collection. Also, advancements in biosensing of human thermoregulation mechanism (e.g., wearable sensors like smartwatches) support the rationale behind the thermal comfort determination. Literature has proposed to link such models with heating, ventilation, and air conditioning (HVAC) systems for operation, which is often called comfort-aware HVAC operations. Also, the use of personal comfort systems (PCSs; e.g., portable heaters) has drawn attention – given their low-energy consumption and capability of creating a microclimate – from Academia.

Spatio-Material

Spatio-material refers to how spaces are created by the materials used in the construction of the space, as well as the materials chosen for the impermanent materials designed to fill those spaces and the aesthetic appeal of both. Assessments include the relationship between positive and negative spaces created by these materials and the materials' intrinsic properties. How a space is designed can affect the health and wellbeing in populations, often connecting to some of the measures discussed previously including light and sound.

Basic parameters of materials and space may be considered, which include the positioning of walls or ceilings to create spaces in which individuals live and work. At the most basic level, these livable and workable spaces impact wellbeing as defined by the ability to perform the defined function necessary for the space (e.g., patient care). This is a basic level of assessment where measurements of space may be tied to the needs of the space and the number of people using the space. For instance, the cubic meters of the home or the number of livable rooms may be compared to the number of people living or working in the space to arrive at a number of people per room or cubic meter per person. Both of these provide insight in the wellbeing of the occupants. This concept can be extended to urban environments with the assessments of kilometers of sidewalks, roads, and parks (open spaces) as contrasted by the footprint of buildings, homes, and other structures incorporated into the urban plan.

This assessment can be taken a step further from individual spaces (e.g., individual rooms) to the interconnectivity between the various spaces, which can provide information on ease of movement and increased functionality. Spaces can also be assessed in terms of volumes or the three-dimensional space in the room or location. The impact of tall ceilings can dramatically increase the volume of a room with the same floor space, providing an impression of more space and changes to wellbeing due to the impact the amount of light, acoustics, and air quality within the space.

Related to volumes is the concept of views or vantage point through a window or the visibility within a city. Rooms with views to the outside give the impression of a larger space even though the finite space with the room does not change. This can be measured by the number of windows with views and the quality of those views. Views into green space have been shown to improve human health and wellbeing over those into urban/concrete landscapes (Astell-Burt & Feng, 2019). This too can be extended to the outdoor environment, where the visibility across the cityscape can change based on the density, the height of buildings or other structures, and the occurrence of open spaces.

In addition to the physical confines of the space, the arrangement of non-permanent materials within those spaces can also have an effect on health and wellbeing. The quantity, placement, and type of these materials (e.g., cubical partitions, seating) can affect the amount of physical space within the room, impacting ease of movement through the space and use for its desired function, and the general aesthetics of the space. Additionally, materials within the space can also affect the light, acoustics, temperature, and air flow within the space, the impact of which can be measured using the techniques highlighted above in the relevant sections.

References

Arenas, J., & Crocker, M. (2010). Recent trends in porous sound-absorbing materials. *Sound & Vibration, 44*(7), 12–18.

Astell-Burt, T., & Feng, X. (2019). Association of urban green space with mental health and general health among adults in Australia. *JAMA Network Open, 2*(7), e198209. https://doi.org/10.1001/jamanetworkopen.2019.8209

Bonnefoy, X. (2007). Inadequate housing and health: An overview. *International Journal of Environment and Pollution, 30*(3–4), 411–429.

Chauvin, J., Pauls, J., & Strobl, L. (2016). Building codes: An often overlooked determinant of health. *Journal of Public Health Policy, 37*(2), 136–148.

de Dear, R., & Brager, G. (1998). Developing an adaptive model of thermal comfort and preference. *ASHRAE Transactions, 104*(1), 145–167.

Donald, I., & Siu, O. L. (2001). Moderating the stress impact of environmental conditions: The effect of organizational commitment in Hong Kong and China. *Journal of Environmental Psychology, 21*(4), 353–368.

Evans, G. W. (2003). The built environment and mental health. *Journal of Urban Health, 80*(4), 536–555.

Fang, L., Wyon, D., Clausen, G., & Fanger, P. (2004). Impact of indoor air temperature and humidity in an office on perceived air quality, SBS symptoms and performance. *Indoor Air, 14*(7), 74–81.

Fanger, P. O. (1967). Calculation of thermal comfort: Introduction of a basic comfort information. *ASHRAE Transactions, 73*, III4.1–III4.20.

Frank, L. D., & Engelke, P. O. (2001). The built environment and human activity patterns: Exploring the impacts of urban form on public health. *Journal of Planning Literature, 16*(2), 202–218.

Galea, S., Ahern, J., Rudenstine, S., Wallace, Z., & Vlahov, D. (2005). Urban built environment and depression: A multilevel analysis. *Journal of Epidemiology & Community Health, 59*(10), 822–827.

Handy, S. L., Boarnet, M. G., Ewing, R., & Killingsworth, R. E. (2002). How the built environment affects physical activity: Views from urban planning. *American Journal of Preventive Medicine, 23*(2), 64–73.

Harris, R. (2015). The changing nature of the workplace and the future of office space. *Journal of Property Investment & Finance, 33*(5), 424–435.

Heerwagen, J. H. (1998, March). Design, productivity and wellbeing: What are the links. In *AIA Conference on Highly Effective Facilities*. Cincinnati, OH.

Jazizadeh, F., Ghahramani, A., Becerik-Gerber, B., Kichkaylo, T., & Orosz, M. (2014). Human-building interaction framework for personalized thermal comfort-driven systems in office buildings. *Journal of Computing in Civil Engineering, 28*(1), 2–16.

Jerdan, S. W., Grindle, M., van Woerden, H. C., & Boulos, M. N. K. (2018). Head-mounted virtual reality and mental health: Critical review of current research. *JMIR Serious Games, 6*(3), e14.

Jung, W., & Jazizadeh, F. (2018). Personalized thermal comfort inference using RGB video images for distributed HVAC control. *Applied Energy, 220,* 829–841.

Kemp, I., Leidelmeijer, K., Marsman, G., & de Hollander, A. (2003). Urban environmental quality and human wellbeing: Towards a conceptual framework and demarcation of concepts; a literature review. *Landscape and Urban Planning, 65*(1–2), 5–18.

Kochtitzky, C., Frumkin, H., Rodriguez, R., Dannenberg, A. L., Rayman, J., Rose, K., … Kanter, T. (2006). Urban planning and public health at CDC. Retrieved from https://www.cdc.gov/mmwr/preview/mmwrhtml/su5502a12.htm

Kopec, D. A. (2006). *Environmental psychology for design.* New York: Fairchild.

Krieger, J., & Higgins, D. L. (2002). Housing and health: Time again for public health action. *American Journal of Public Health, 92*(5), 758–768.

Kyttä, A., Broberg, A., & Kahila, M. (2012). Urban environment and children's active lifestyle: SoftGIS revealing children's behavioral patterns and meaningful places. *American Journal of Health Promotion, 26*(5), e137–e148.

Lamb, S., & Kwok, K. (2015). A longitudinal investigation of work environment stressors on the performance and wellbeing of office workers. *Applied Ergonomics, 52,* 104.

Lee, P., & Jeon, J. (2013). Relating traffic, construction, and ventilation noise to cognitive performances and subjective perceptions. *The Journal of the Acoustical Society of America, 134*(4), 2765–2772.

Leung, D. (2015). Outdoor-indoor air pollution in urban environment: Challenges and opportunity. *Frontiers in Environmental Science, 2,* 69.

Ličina, F., et al. (2018). Development of the ASHRAE Global thermal comfort Database II. *Building and Environment, 142,* 502–512.

Maples-Keller, J., Bunnell, B., Kim, S., & Rothbaum, B. (2017). The use of virtual reality technology in treatment of anxiety and other psychiatric disorders. *Harvard Review of Psychiatry, 25*(3), 103–113.

Marion, M. (2003). *Guidance of young children* (6th ed.). Upper Saddle River, NJ: Prentice Hall.

McAllister, J. (2014). Four ways virtual reality can help us design and create better health care facilities. Retrieved from https://www.beckershospitalreview.com/healthcare-information-technology/four-ways-virtual-reality-can-help-us-design-and-create-better-healthcare-facilities.html

Melrose, S. (2015). Seasonal Affective Disorder: An Overview of Assessment and Treatment Approaches. *Depression research and treatment, 2015,* 178564. https://doi.org/10.1155/2015/178564. https://www.ncbi.nlm.nih.gov/pmc/articles/PMC4673349/

National Research Council. (1981). *Indoor pollutants.* National Academies

O'Hara, S., Klar, R. T., Patterson, E. S., Morris, N. S., Ascenzi, J., Fackler, J. C., & Perry, D. J. (2018). Macrocognition in the healthcare built environment (mHCBE): A focused ethnographic study of "neighborhoods" in a pediatric intensive care unit. *HERD: Health Environments Research & Design Journal, 11*(2), 104–123.

Rashmi, M., Kasthuri, A., & Rodrigues, R. (2016). Senior friendly hospitals: Development and application of criteria: A descriptive study. *Indian Journal of Community Medicine, 41*(4), 256–262.

Rizzo, A. (2003). A SWOT analysis of the field of virtual rehabilitation. In *Proceedings of the Second International Workshop on Virtual Rehabilitation* (pp. 1–2).

Saratsis, E., Dogan, T., & Reinhart, C. (2016). Simulation-based daylighting analysis procedure for developing urban zoning rules. *Building Research & Information, 45*(5), 478–491

Srivastava, K., Das, R. C., & Chaudhury, S. (2014). Virtual reality applications in mental health: Challenges and perspectives. *Industrial Psychiatry Journal, 23*(2), 83.

Tambs, K. (2004). Moderate effects of hearing loss on mental health and subjective wellbeing: Results from the Nord-Trøndelag hearing loss study. *Psychosomatic Medicine, 65*(5), 776–782.

Taylor, S., & Hugentobler, W. (2016). Is low indoor humidity a driver for healthcare-associated infections? Retrieved from https://www.condair.com/m/0/poster-taylor-hugentobler-gent-indoor-air-2016.pdf

Ulrich RS, Zimring C, Zhu X, et al. A Review of the Research Literature on Evidence-Based Healthcare Design. *HERD: Health Environments Research & Design Journal.* 2008;1(3):61–125. doi:10.1177/193758670800100306. https://journals.sagepub.com/doi/10.1177/193758670800100306

Urban Land Institute, McCormick, K., MacCleery, R., & Hammerschmidt, S. (2013). *Intersections: Health and the built environment.* Urban Land Institute, Building Healthy Places Initiative.

Wolkoff, P. (2018). Indoor air humidity, air quality, and health – an overview. *International Journal of Hygiene and Environmental Health, 221*(3), 376–390.

World Health Organization. (2018). WHO housing and health guidelines. Retrieved from https://www.who.int/sustainable-development/publications/housing-health-guidelines/en/.

3   Material Measures

Materials

The built environment is characterized by the materials that comprise its spatial configurations. There are numerous materials utilized in building construction, which may vary depending upon the regional resources and methods or depending upon the building program needs and budget. This chapter introduces the major material groups based on chemistry and physical characteristics. The influence of material extraction, manufacturing, and compositions on environmental health is presented by addressing built environment applications. The information in this chapter provides the fundamentals for understanding the characteristics of materials and why it is necessary to reframe the selection of materials for buildings through consideration of environmental and human health measures.

Material Groups

There are seven major material groups based on the chemical and physical structure characteristics, including nontechnical ceramics, technical ceramics, metals, natural materials, polymers and elastomers, foams, and composites (Figure 3.1). The nature of chemical bonds and physical microstructures of each material group demonstrates specific characteristics that define distinct performance properties in application. In addition to the material chemistry, the resource extraction, manufacturing processes, construction processes, and demolition of building materials also impact both environmental and human health.

Nontechnical Ceramics

Nontechnical ceramics include materials such as stone, masonry, concrete, and earthen materials. These ceramics have a high compressive strength and are used as building materials for this purpose as well as for interior finishing elements. The nontechnical ceramics are typically benign in their constructed

DOI: 10.4324/9780367814748-5

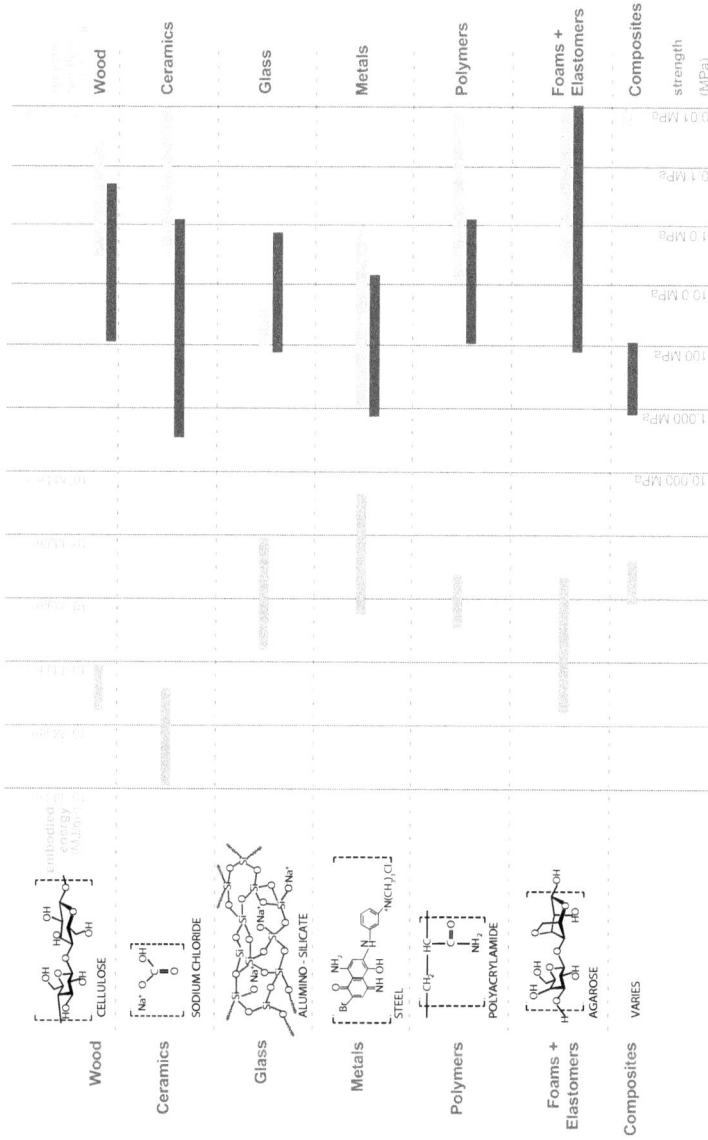

Figure 3.1 Composite Diagram: Material Scanning Electron Microscope (SEM) Images and Chemical Notations of Basic Material Groups.

context and comprise the oldest and longest remaining buildings from ancient eras all around the world. Some of the earliest building techniques using rammed earth and adobe sun-dried masonry block construction prove to be the lowest environmental impact to this day (Ciancio et al., 2015). Unlike contemporary masonry and concrete construction techniques, which require high amounts of heat energy for curing or release large amounts of carbon dioxide, the rammed earth and adobe processes are environmentally clean. Some adobe construction methods incorporate straw to enhance curing consistencies; however, there are possible health drawbacks with resulting mildew and fungi growth in such modules (Pacheco-Torgal & Jalali, 2012).

Some additional properties of nontechnical ceramic construction that provide human health benefits include the high thermal capacitance or thermal inertia that encourages stabilized indoor comfort temperatures. In addition, the thickness of the earthen material construction provides some noise reduction between outdoor and indoor spaces. Furthermore, for earthen materials such as adobe or rammed earth in particular, the exposed ceramic is serving as a hygroscopic condition providing a balancing effect for indoor relative humidity that results in human health benefits (Cobîrzan et al., 2016). In some cases, the use of salts and minerals for the ceramic construction material may be implemented, which provides improved air quality due to the ionization effects (Chervinskaya & Zilber, 1995; Hedman et al., 2006; Horowitz, 2010).

Stone quarrying and earthen material extraction processes can also be environmentally problematic due to the production of stone dusts in the quarry processing, which result in airborne particulates that can negatively impact human and animal life (Sheikh et al., 2011). The transport of fired masonry or concrete masonry units (CMUs) from manufacturing locations or of natural stone from quarry-pit origin, to building sites is typically of very long distances and results in greenhouse gas (GHG) emissions from the transportation mode.

Emerging processes for fabricating masonry building materials incorporate biological chemistry principles and microorganisms that aid in the curing process so that heat energy input and carbon emissions are eliminated altogether (Soleimani-Dashtaki et al., 2017). Cementitious building products that are grown using microorganisms alleviate the need for firing due to the biologically controlled curing process.

Technical Ceramics

Technical ceramics includes materials such as glass. Glass materials have an amorphous bonding pattern due to the high amount of heat energy input during the manufacturing process. In its solid state, glass is environmentally benign and resistant to degradation. Glass provides numerous health benefits for building occupants because of both natural daylight transmittance and transparency for views outward to nature (Sadar, 2008).

Advancements of glazing technologies for buildings is a vast market. Numerous types of spectrally selective coatings are developed for glazing applications to manage the solar spectrum transmittance conditions. Some coatings prevent ultraviolet (UV) light from entering, protecting humans from harmful electromagnetic rays. Other coatings focus on short-wave infrared (IR) radiation to alleviate heat gain inside buildings, helping to maintain thermally comfortable temperatures for occupants.

The recyclability of glass allows for reduced environmental impact of the material since from extraction and deployment in application; the material can be melted and repurposed for new use through multiple life cycles. The intense heat energy required for manufacturing glass, and the resulting carbon emissions, is the primary environmental challenge with technical ceramic building products. Transportation modes for moving glass building products from the manufacturing plant to the construction site also have an environmental impact to be considered on a case-by-case basis dependent on volume or weight, distance, and transport method. Because of the fragility and brittleness of glass, a large amount of packing material is required to protect the products, contributing to additional environmental impact through foams and plastic waste.

Metals

Metals include a range of materials such as steel, aluminum, copper, titanium, and other metal alloys. The chemical bonding structure of metals is defined by the free electrons at outer valence rings, which provides for the high thermal conductivity as well as the ductility associated with these materials that allows for reversibility between liquid and solid states. The most challenging environmental aspect of metals is the mining extraction processes, which tend to leave residual metals in the mine tailings at extraction sites that leach into surface and groundwater and create exposures through windblown dust (Nuss & Eckelman, 2014). Furthermore, the amount of energy and water required to conduct mining activities is extremely high (Mavis, 2003).

When metal products are integrated in buildings, those exposed to the outdoor elements may have corrosive interactions with water and moisture over time that lend to problematic leaching of metal particulates into air, soil, and surface- and groundwater sources (Leygraf et al., 2016; Mcalister et al., 2008). The distribution of leached metal particulates into soil and water systems impacts ecological health and ultimately finds its way back to humans, impacting agricultural and aquaculture food sources through problematic bioaccumulation.

Recyclability of metals is well established, in part due to the large quantities of metals used in modern society, and in part because of the value of metal materials, both necessitating the development of recycling techniques and processes to be established. Metals are relatively easily recyclable because of the ease in re-melting and re-forming with heat energy. The environmental impact of transporting metal building products from the manufacturing plant to the construction site can be quite large due to the heavy weight of most metal products.

Natural Materials

Natural materials include renewable resources such as wood, cork, and bamboo. They exhibit a range of polymeric bonding patterns that provide for unique properties with anisotropic strength and thermal resistance. They tend to have low overall environmental impact since the resources are renewable and do not necessarily require additional processing, other than cutting and shaping, after source extraction. The natural materials that impact human health are those which are composited with adhesives and binders, such as laminates and pressed fiber boards, that result in problematic volatile organic compounds (VOCs) being released in indoor environments (Ebnesajjad, 2011).

Natural materials integrated in buildings may provide human health benefits with visual aspects of warmth and references to natural settings, shown to be beneficial for human neurology (Mcgee & Marshall-Baker, 2015). Certain natural materials, such as cork, will also enhance the acoustic environment due to the air-filled material structure that allows for sound absorption. One of the human health challenges with natural materials in buildings is that these materials are a food source for certain microbes, molds, and insects, and thus can negatively affect the air quality or the perceived health of the building.

Polymers and Elastomers

Polymers and elastomers are synthesized materials that exhibit ductile properties due to the long-chain monomer repeatable cross-linking. This material group is considered one of the most problematic for environmental and human health. Many of a building's interior finishes, such as paints and carpets and furnishings, are comprised of polymers. Such elements may contribute to sick building syndrome (SBS) if they are laden with VOCs and the release of ultrafine particles that are problematic for the human respiratory system (Spengler et al., 2001). Many polymers and elastomers also tend to be chemically synthesized with covalent bonds that are very difficult to break down and prevent recyclability; thus, the life cycle of such materials is limited, while the embodied energy for single use is already very high.

Advancements in polymer science and biotechnology are lending to numerous emerging options for biocompatible polymer materials (Habibi & Lucia, 2012). However, in general, the environmentally healthy polymers will be those that have weaker bonds, which result in lower thermal and mechanical stability in comparison with covalently bonded polymers. While such polymer products can be more readily recycled, they also degrade more easily and may lend to a shorter life span in building applications.

Foams

Foams are related to polymers with repeated long-chain monomer cross-links but vary in the macrostructure, which is highly porous with either regular or irregular open-cell and closed-cell patterns. In building applications, foams provide a number of human health benefits, such as thermal control of indoor environments due to the high thermal resistance values, as well as noise control due to the enhanced sound absorption properties. The process of applying particular building insulation foams can be very damaging to the environment due to the airborne contaminants that result from spray-foam processes with products such as polyurethane (Naldzhiev et al., 2017), a chemically cross-linked thermoset that cannot be easily recycled at end of life. Some of the blowing agents used for the spray-foam process contribute to stratospheric ozone depletion, such as trichlorofluoromethane and other chlorine-based agents (Shankland, 1990).

Historically, many foam-based building insulation products also contain other contaminants that are hazardous for environmental and human health. Examples include Tris(1-chloro-2-propyl) phosphate (TCPP) is primarily used as a flame retardant in rigid and flexible polyurethane foam and hexabromocyclododecane (HBCD), which are highly toxic flame retardants and insecticides used in products such as polyisocyanurate and expanded polystyrene insulation (Vo et al., 2011). Such chemicals can leach into occupied building spaces over time due to airborne insulation dust particles or into soils and groundwater for below-grade insulation installations. Many foam products for buildings have also incorporated elements that are both carcinogens and asthmagens, including formaldehyde, boric acid, persistent, bioaccumulative, and toxic (PBT) impurities, and problematic dedusting oils.

Emerging building insulation foams eliminate harmful toxins in both the chemical composition and the application process. Bioinspired foams are also advancing towards the building product market, such as mycelium-based foams sustainably grown with fungus biofabrication techniques. Other building foam alternatives utilize by-product waste from the blue-jean industry to make an environmentally clean batt insulation product.

Composites

Composite materials include a wide range of options and continue to expand in material engineering and design for enhanced properties and characteristics.

Some examples of composites used for building materials are carbon fiber-reinforced concrete, polymers, or glass (CFRC, CFRP, or CFRG, respectively). For the environmental and human health impacts of composite material chemistry, reference to the original material groups should be made. The manufacturing of composites often requires some type of heating method or a chemical binder to induce cohesion between dissimilar materials. Composite materials can be environmentally problematic at end of life due to the challenges for separating the compound materials into respective purities required for reuse (Biron, 2013).

Material Chemistry

The range of material conditions that influence human health and wellbeing include thermal, visual, acoustic, haptic, and noxious aspects. The chemistry and microstructures of materials ultimately define these characteristics that impact human perception and health. The phenomenological conditions of materials that influence human sensing and perception are addressed in Chapter 2.2. Of significance to the material chemistry, manufacturing, and building applications are metrics related to the embodied energy, strength, and durability, as well as the end-of-life recycle fraction (Figure 3.1).

Contemporary building design practice standards include rubrics that address environmental and health ethics through material specifications (Bergman, 2012). Examples of such standards are found in the US Green Building Council (USGBC) Leadership in Energy and Environmental Design (LEED) rating systems, the Living Building Challenge (LBC) Red List and Declare Label systems, and the WELL Building Standard. The American Society for Testing and Materials (ASTM) establishes the protocols and procedures for ensuring certain qualitative and quantitative standards are established for materials that will be deployed in building applications. Environmental toxicology of building materials is one aspect that may be addressed by ASTM methods for specific products, but the primary focus for ASTM is with installation and structural strength guidelines. National initiatives to incentivize change in the building industry material practices to improve human and environmental health include Housing and Urban Development (HUD)'s Healthy Homes program and the US Environmental Protection Agency's (USEPA) Sustainable Materials Management (SMM) program.

High-performance building practices and architecture firms with research initiatives are implementing integrated sensing with the material systems of buildings during construction and operation in order to monitor ongoing performance measures. The Dynamic Plaque system connected with the LEED rating is managed by Arc Skoru and integrated real-time metrics on building performance in accordance with the LEED categories (Arc Skoru, 2023). The Philadelphia-based architecture practice of Kieran-Timberlake (KT) integrates data sensing techniques in pre- and post-occupancy design projects, and ultimately developed the Pointelist building sensing network start-up through their KT Innovations research arm (KT, 2022). Many of the sensing modes with these practices address material performance through air quality, thermal, and moisture management monitoring. Advancements in material technologies exhibit direct integration of embedded fiber optics allowing for the ability to sense electromagnetic changes indicating potentially problematic microbe and moisture developments in early stages (Arhant et al., 2018).

Ultimately, the understanding of material chemistry and environmental and human toxicology provides a strong basis for scrutinizing modern building material manufacturing, installation, and specification processes and standards. Because the construction industry and building product manufacturing processes are deeply engrained with expectations for material performance based on methods with unacceptable chemistry and emissions, innovations and change in this area are slow to evolve, yet beginning to occur. The ongoing sensing and monitoring of building materials and spaces in both pre- and post-occupancy stages of construction and operation assist with foundational evidence on environmental and human health measures. Through education of next-generation practitioners in the architecture and engineering fields, and through policy and regulation modifications, expectations for healthy building materials and environmentally sound manufacturing and application will persevere.

Smart Materials

Smart materials are those that sense and react to environmental signals or stimuli, which can include mechanical, magnetic, or chemical signals.

Piezoelectric materials are a group of smart materials that produce a voltage when mechanical stressed is applied to the material. These materials can be incorporated into structural construction materials like concrete and can act as a sensor by creating an electric field. For example, PZT (lead zirconium titanate) ceramics can be embedded in concrete to create a material that is capable of sensing structural deficiencies in buildings, alerting engineers to potential threats to human health (Chen et al., 2019). Additionally, piezoelectric carbon fibers are also a common additive into asphalt concrete on roadways. The addition of this material allows the roadways to be used as traffic recording sensors as the stress of each vehicle moves across the surface, informing vehicle health and safety concerns. These sensors also have the capability of changing mechanical energy to electrical energy created by the traffic, and this can be used as a source of energy (Yu et al., 2023). This type of smart concrete is also used to improve the safety of sidewalks and bridges in ice-prone areas either passively due to thermal properties compared to traditional materials or actively when an electric current is applied.

Other group of smart building materials are those that incorporate aerogels or hydrogels into their structures. These gels are comprised of a three-dimensional framework of polymers with an internal medium of either air (aerogels) or a liquid (hydrogels). These materials are particularly resistant to heat and cold and are often used for insulation and temperature control within building systems. Additionally, use of these gels reduces material weight and aero and hydrogels considered more environmentally sustainable than other conventional options. These materials also provide fire protection and are effective acoustic dampeners, reduce the acoustic vibrations from external noise pollution. An example are hydroceramics that incorporate hydrogels into their structure and are capable of retaining 500 times their volume in water. They are effective moisture-thermal insulators absorbing moisture in high humidity and releasing it during hot, dry periods to cool the local environment (Peeks & Badarnah, 2021). These materials can be used to improve the efficiency of buildings and human comfort within the built environment.

Shape memory materials (SMMs) are another class of smart materials that have the capability of deforming under various stressors, but when the stress is removed, the material reverts back to its original shape. SMMs often include super elastic metal alloys such as nickel-titanium or viscoelasticity polymers. The materials are excellent for structures built in seismically active zones and those with severe weather patterns including hurricanes. Similarly, magneto-restrictive materials are SMMs that are sensitive to and change shape in magnetic fields. These materials are also used in high-impact environments as shock absorbers as well as host of structural engineering applications. Magneto- and electro-rheological fluids are materials that change shape and viscosity when controlled by their respective magnetic or electrical fields (Bahl et al., 2020). These materials have similar uses to SMMs including shock absorption and vibration suppression and are integral in large-scale construction within the built environment.

Chromoactive smart materials change color with an external stimulus such as temperature (thermochromic) or light (photochromic). These materials can be integrated into a building's design to improve human health and wellbeing through visual stimuli. For example, external facades or internal wallpaper can change color depending on the stimulus to optimize the color of the room or control the amount of light entering a space. Smart glass (electrochromic) employs a similar function to thermo- and photochromic smart materials but operates through the use of electrical current and thin nanocoating on the glass. The material adapts to changing outdoor conditions and controls the amount of radiation entering the room to improve health and wellbeing, as well as reduce energy costs (Nguyen et al., 2020). Various smart coatings, similar to the thin film on smart glass, also exist for internal and external building uses. These include materials that contain titanium dioxide nanoparticles, which are effective at increasing chemical reactions when exposed to light (photocatalysis). These help to remove dirt and microbes from surfaces

(Padmanabhan & John, 2020). As a result, these materials are effective at odor control and improve the air quality of indoor environments. When used externally, there is a cost savings associated with a longer duration of time before exterior maintenance and cleaning is required.

References

Arc Skoru. (2023). Arc for LEED, Performance-based green building certification. Retrieved from https://arcskoru.com/arc-for-leed

Arhant, M., Meek, N., Penumadu, D., et al. (2018). Residual strains using integrated continuous fiber optic sensing in thermoplastic composites and structural health monitoring. *Experimental Mechanicals, 58*, 167–176. https://doi.org/10.1007/s11340-017-0339-2

Bahl, S., Nagar, H., Singh, I., & Sehgal, S. (2020). Smart materials types, properties and applications: A review. https://www.sciencedirect.com/science/article/abs/pii/S2214785320331278. Materials Today: Proceedings, *28*, 1302–1306

Bergman. (2012). *Sustainable design: A critical guide* (1st ed.). Princeton Architectural Press. Princeton Architectural Press New York, NY.

Biron, M. (2013). *Thermosets and composites: Material selection, applications, manufacturing and cost analysis.* Elsevier, Amsterdam.

Chen, J., Qiu, Q., Han, Y., & Lau, D. (2019). Piezoelectric materials for sustainable building structures: Fundamentals and applications. *Renewable & Sustainable Energy Reviews, 101*, 14–25. https://doi.org/10.1016/j.rser.2018.09.038

Chervinskaya, A. V., & Zilber, N. A. (1995). Halotherapy for treatment of respiratory diseases. *Journal of Aerosol Medicine: The Official Journal of the International Society for Aerosols in Medicine, 8*(3), 221–232. https://doi.org/10.1089/jam.1995.8.221

Ciancio, D., Beckett, C., Augarde, C., & Jaquin, P. (2015). First international conference on rammed earth construction: Report. *Proceedings of the Institution of Civil Engineers-Construction Materials, 169*(5), 271–275. https://doi.org/10.1680/jcoma.15.00038

Cobîrzan, Balog, A.-A., Belean, B., Borodi, G., Dădârlat, D., & Streza, M. (2016). Thermophysical properties of masonry units: Accurate characterization by means of photothermal techniques and relationship to porosity and mineral composition. *Construction & Building Materials, 105*, 297–306. https://doi.org/10.1016/j.conbuildmat.2015.12.056

Ebnesajjad, S. (2011). *Handbook of Adhesives and Surface Preparation.* Ebnesajjad, S. (ed), pp. 137–183, William Andrew Publishing, Oxford.

Habibi, & Lucia, L. A. (2012). *Polysaccharide building blocks: A sustainable approach to the development of renewable biomaterials* (1. Aufl.), Hoboken, NJ. Wiley. https://doi.org/10.1002/9781118229484

Hedman, J., Hugg, T., Sandell, J., & Haahtela, T. (2006). The effect of salt chamber treatment on bronchial hyperresponsiveness in asthmatics. *Allergy, 61*(5), 605–610. https://doi.org/10.1111/j.1398-9995.2006.01073.x

Horowitz, S. (2010). Salt cave therapy: Rediscovering the benefits of an old preservative. *Alternative and Complementary Therapies, 16*(3), 158–162.

KieranTimberlake (KT). (2022). Pointelist. Retrieved from https://www.pointelist.com/

Leygraf, C., Wallinder, I. O., Tidblad, J. & Graedel, T. (2016). *Atmospheric Corrosion.* John Wiley & Sons, Inc., Hoboken, New Jersey. https://doi.org/10.1002/9781118762134

Mavis, J. (2003). *Water use in industries of the future: Mining industry. Industrial water management: A systems approach* (2nd ed.). Prepared by CH2M HILL for the Center for Waste Reduction Technologies, American Institute of Chemical Engineers, New York.

McAlister, Smith, B. J., & Török, A. (2008). Transition metals and water-soluble ions in deposits on a building and their potential catalysis of stone decay. *Atmospheric Environment (1994)*, *42*(33), 7657–7668. https://doi.org/10.1016/j.atmosenv.2008.05.067

McGee, B., & Marshall-Baker, A. (2015). Loving nature from the inside out: A biophilia matrix identification strategy for designers. *HERD: Health Environments Research & Design Journal, 8*(4), 115–130. https://doi.org/10.1177/1937586715578644

Naldzhiev, D., Mumovic, D., & Strlič, M. (2017). Method development for measuring volatile organic compound (VOC) emission rates from spray foam insulation (SPF) and their interrelationship with indoor air quality (IAQ), human health and ventilation strategies. *Conference: 38th AIVC – 6th TightVent & 4th Venticool Conference, 2017 Ventilating Healthy Low-Energy Buildings.* Nottingham, United Kingdom.

Nguyen, T. D., Yeo, L. P., Ong, A. J., Zhiwei, W., Mandler, D., Magdassi, S., & Tok, A. I. Y. (2020). Electrochromic smart glass coating on functional nano-frameworks for effective building energy conservation. *Materials Today Energy, 18*, 100496. https://doi.org/10.1016/j.mtener.2020.100496

Nuss, & Eckelman, M. J. (2014). Life cycle assessment of metals: A scientific synthesis. *PloS One, 9*(7), e101298–e101298. https://doi.org/10.1371/journal.pone.0101298

Pacheco-Torgal, F., & Jalali, S. (2012) Earth construction: Lessons from the past for future eco-efficient construction. *Construction and Building Materials, 29*, 512–519. https://doi.org/10.1016/j.conbuildmat.2011.10.054

Padmanabhan, N. T., & John, H. (2020). Titanium dioxide based self-cleaning smart surfaces: A short review. *Journal of Environmental Chemical Engineering, 8*(5), 104211. https://doi.org/10.1016/j.jece.2020.104211

Peeks, M., & Badarnah, L. (2021). Textured building facades: Utilizing morphological adaptations found in nature for evaporative cooling. *Biomimetics (Basel, Switzerland), 6*(2), 24. https://doi.org/10.3390/biomimetics6020024

Sadar. (2008). The healthful ambience of Vitaglass: Light, glass and the curative environment. *Arq (London, England), 12*(3–4), 269–281. https://doi.org/10.1017/S1359135508001206

Shankland, I. (1990) CFC alternatives for thermal insulation foams. *International Journal of Refrigeration, 13*, 113–121. https://doi.org/10.1016/0140-7007(90)90010-T

Sheikh, A., Rana, S. V., & Pal, A. K. (2011). Environmental health assessment of stone crushers in and around Jhansi, U. P., India. *Journal of Ecophysiology and Occupational Health, 11*, 107–115.

Soleimani-Dashtaki, Ventura, C. E., & Banthia, N. (2017). Seismic strengthening of unreinforced masonry walls using sprayable eco-friendly ductile cementitious composite (EDCC). *Procedia Engineering, 210*, 154–164. https://doi.org/10.1016/j.proeng.2017.11.061

Spengler, J. D., MDMS, J. M. S., & DCIH, J. F. M. S. (2001). *Indoor air quality handbook.* McGraw-Hill Education, New York, NY.

Vo, C. V., Bunge, F., Duffy, J., & Hood, L. (2011). Advances in thermal insulation of extruded polystyrene foams. *Cellular Polymers, 30*(3), 137–156. http://doi.org/10.1177/026248931103000303

Yu, Y., Shi, Y., Kurita, H., Jia, Y., Wang, Z., & Narita, F. (2023). Carbon fiber-reinforced piezoelectric nanocomposites: Design, fabrication and evaluation for damage detection and energy harvesting. *Composites. Part A, Applied Science and Manufacturing, 172*, 107587. https://doi.org/10.1016/j.compositesa.2023.107587

Part II

Methods

Measurement Techniques, Tools, and Methods for Health and Wellbeing

4 Sensing and Data Acquisition

Introduction

The basics of sensing and data acquisition in built environments and human biosensing are discussed in this chapter. The range of sensing techniques covered includes environmental sensing, participatory sensing, biosensing, neurosensing, material sensing, and microbial sensing (Figure 4.1). The types of data collected from sensing devices are discussed in terms of the various quantifiable and qualifiable metrics that can be associated with the different sets, resolutions, and scales of information. In addition to the human, environmental, and material data acquisition and management, additional data that might be needed for related calculations, such as construction costs for return-on-investment (ROI) analysis, are discussed.

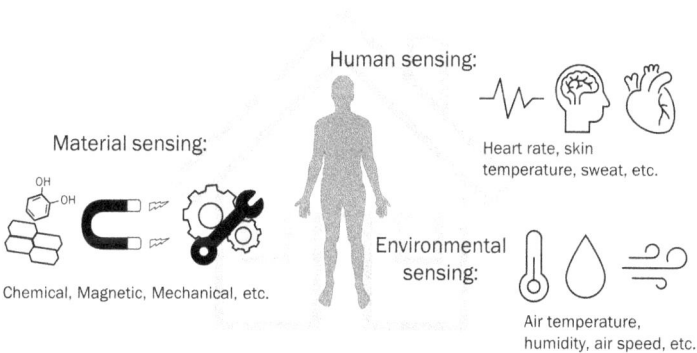

Human sensing:
Heart rate, skin temperature, sweat, etc.

Material sensing:
Chemical, Magnetic, Mechanical, etc.

Environmental sensing:
Air temperature, humidity, air speed, etc.

Figure 4.1 Composite Diagram: Interscalar Environmental, Material, and Human Sensing Variable.

DOI: 10.4324/9780367814748-7

Sensing Techniques

When considering the wide range of variables between the built environment and human health, a plethora of sensing information can be considered. There are many ways to collect data from the built environment and from humans, including observations and surveys. However, the primary focus in this chapter is the collection of data by means of sensing technologies and methods. The use of sensors provides a focus for data collection that typically results in reliable, accurate, and unbiased information when compiled into holistic datasets. The interpretation and analysis of the larger datasets can be accomplished by the individual researcher or by computational means.

Environmental Sensing

Humans are situated in their environments in multidimensional ways, all of which comprise individual or collective environmental attributes that in turn play a role in health and wellbeing outcomes. While some may only consider their immediate physical environment to be their entire environment, it is important to remember the multidimensional aspects of the total environment, all of which influence human health. According to the World Health Organization (WHO), in the context of health, the total environment includes its physical, natural, social, and behavioral attributes (Prüss-stün & Corvalán, 2006).

Since human health is defined by a variety of factors, it is important to utilize available sensing technologies to objectively measure and determine potential barriers or facilitators to health and wellness in individual or communal spaces. There are a wide variety of sensors available today that are employed to measure air quality, soil moisture, water quality, and the quantity and quality of light in different environments. Two important environmental attributes that are discussed in this section are air quality and light. Acoustics or noise levels, thermal comfort, water quality, and spatio-material measures, however, are also factors influencing the wellbeing of individuals inhabiting a built environment, which can be measured with sensing technologies. Additionally, many sensing technologies have the capability to provide real-time and continuous data collection. This feature is valuable, since we typically perform a number of different tasks throughout the day as well as undergo physiological changes as a result of these tasks, environmental conditions, and other personal factors. It is, therefore, important to measure physical, physiological, psychological, and environmental conditions simultaneously and continuously, and analyze how all these factors collectively impact individual health and wellbeing.

Air quality is an important aspect of the environment which impacts all community members in an outdoor or indoor environment. Indoor air quality, commonly referred to as IAQ, or outdoor air quality depends upon a variety of factors. To measure the effects of air pollution and effectively use and interpret data obtained from environmental sensors, it is important to understand the types of air pollution in the environment that sensors try to measure and quantify. The two main types are those which naturally occur, such as particulate matter (PM), and anthropogenic types of air pollution, which come from sources such as electric plants or vehicles. Since air quality is closely associated with health, environmental sensors focus on common air pollutants in the environment which are most strongly linked to negative health outcomes. Some of the most common ones defined by the US Environmental Protection Agency (USEPA) are ground-level ozone, PM, nitrogen dioxide (NO_2), carbon monoxide (CO), sulfur dioxide (SO_2), and lead (USEPA, 2019). The USEPA regulates the levels of these common air pollutants to ensure that typical human exposure to them in the environment complies with certain standards. These standards were defined following the Clean Air Act, which required the production of the National Ambient Air Quality Standards (NAAQS) (USEPA, 2016a, 2016b).

To further understand air quality measurements, it is important to understand all the units used to measure different types of air pollutants. For the common air pollutants, sometimes referred to as "criteria" air pollutants, measurements are usually made in parts per million (ppm), parts per billion (ppb), or micrograms per cubic meter of air ($\mu g/m^3$), depending on the pollutant, how harmful it is, or the measured length of time of the exposure. For example, carbon monoxide (CO) should not exceed 9 ppm over the course of 8 hours or may exceed 35 ppm over 1 hour on only one occasion per year, while lead exposures should never exceed 0.15 $\mu g/m^3$ every three months as per the USEPA (2016b). The maximum level of lead exposure, however, was much higher at 1.5 $\mu g/m^3$ prior to it being lowered to the current standard in 2008 (USEPA, 2016b). Nitrogen dioxide's (NO_2) should not exceed 53 ppb in any given year. Ground-level ozone exposure is not allowed to exceed 0.070 ppm over 8 hours, with sulfur dioxide (SO_2) having a much higher threshold for 1- and 3-hour intervals at 75 ppb and 0.5 ppm, respectively. For PM, exposures are divided into two separate categories based upon the size of the PM, $PM_{2.5}$ (PM sized 2.5 microns) and PM_{10} (PM sized 10 microns). An individual's exposure to $PM_{2.5}$ exposure should never exceed 12–15 $\mu g/m^3$ annually, while for PM_{10}, an exposure of 150 $\mu g/m^3$ has been established as an annual maximum over a 24-hour period (USEPA, 2016a). Lastly, the level of carbon dioxide is often a common measure of indoor air quality due to its contribution to human health. Seppänen et al. (1999) synthesized that the risk of sick building syndrome symptoms (e.g., eye, nose, and throat irritation; skin redness; mental fatigue; headache; nausea and dizziness; etc.) decreased with CO_2 concentrations below 800 ppm. Occupants are the major contributor to the concentration of CO_2, and it is considered as an effective indicator of indoor pollutants given its surrogate role. Hence, the number of occupants in a space is one of the criteria to determine the minimum ventilation rate (ASHRAE 62.1, 2019). Light is another important and quantifiable measure of our environments. When measuring light, the main variables of the light source that need to be considered from a human health perspective are brightness, energy, and wavelength. Watts (W), the most commonly known measure of light, is used to express the amount of energy used in the production of light. Flux is measured in lumens (lm) and is defined as the amount of energy a light emits every second. Another important quantifiable measure which uses lumens in its measurement is lux (lx), or the standard unit of measurement of illuminance. One lux (lx) is equivalent to one lumen (lm) per square meter (m^2), or lm/m^2. While lux is the metric unit of measure illuminance, one foot-candle (fc) is the nonmetric (non-international system of units (non-SI)) unit of illuminance equivalent to one lumen per square foot (ft^2). It also equals 10.764 lux and is used mostly in the United States. The recommended illuminance of a space in lux or foot-candles corresponds to what types of activities are carried out in that particular space (Mikulka, 2018). For example, while a measure of 200 lux would be appropriate for a space with low need for visual acuity like a restroom or dining room, a measure of 500 lux would be more appropriate for a setting like a kitchen which has a higher but still moderate demand for better color judgment or visual acuity (DiLaura et al., 2014).

The brightness of light sources and levels of their different wavelengths has also been found to be closely associated with mood, learning, productivity, and circadian rhythms in humans, that is, the physiological, mental, and behavioral changes that follow a daily cycle including sleeping and waking (LeGates et al., 2014). Different wavelengths of light are measured in nanometers (nm). This data can be measured and collected continuously by sensory devices, which are also available as mobile or wearable types. These devices usually have the ability to measure sleep and activity at the same time, so that all these variables can be studied together to find possible associations – especially between light quality and circadian rhythms.

Sound and noise are also measurable with different tools and devices. Sound meters identify the intensity of propagation wavelengths of phonons emanating from a source to a receptor point in space. The transmission of sound through a medium (air, water, solid materials) is dependent on the decibel emission from the source and the molecular composition of the medium. The noise level, measured in decibels, determines the impact on human hearing and reception of pressure against the ear drum. Sound disperses based on the third power law – Steven's power law – becoming less intense by a factor of one-third each time the distance from the originating source doubles (Irwin & Corballis, 1968).

Temperature is important for thermoregulation of the core body temperature, which should be maintained at 97.7°F–99.5°F (36.5 °C–37.5°C). The temperature of the environment can directly influence both the perception and the physical experience of body temperature change – feeling too hot in the sun and too cold in the snow. With extreme thermal conditions, the body can experience an emergent state of health challenges requiring medical attention – either hyperthermia, when the body is overheated, or hypothermia, when the body experiences loss of function in freezing conditions. The thermal environment is one of the earliest and primary reasons that humans construct shelter and dwellings to protect and mediate from the temperatures that fall outside of both comfort and functional health ranges. Temperature is most strictly defined by dry-bulb temperature (DBT) measures, which are made with DBT sensors. The acceptable human thermal comfort temperature range typically falls between 68°F and 81.5°F (20°C–27.5°C) (Aqilah et al., 2022; ASHRAE, 2020), though this range can shift based on environmental acclimation, age, gender, and physiological, physical, and psychological factors. In addition, the radiant conditions of an environment, when in direct sun or in the path of reflected heat, can drastically shift the thermal experience. There are advancements on basic thermal calculations for human comfort and perception, identified through mean radiant temperature (MRT) and physiological equivalent temperature (PET). Each of these measures consists of a set of variables that contribute to the experienced temperature. MRT is calculated based on the 360-degree environmental and material conditions surrounding a position in space (presumably where a human is standing or sitting). The reflected and emitted radiant heat or cool from all surrounding conditions is taken into account based on two fisheye lens views (depicting 180 degrees each) and analyzed for view factors based on a radial segmented grid projected onto the views. The view factor defines the amount or percentage of influence that a material or environmental spatial condition will have on the human's thermal experience. MRT also takes into account sources of conduction between the human body and direct contact with surfaces. The PET is quite similar and was developed to provide a comparison of outdoor thermal comfort measures compared to those used for indoors that excluded aspects such as radiation. Specific sensors can be used for measuring MRT and PET, such as a black globe thermometer. Emerging trends of sensor types, those which collectively combine the parameters of interest (radiant heat and DBT), are discussed in the next chapter.

Humidity also plays an important role in both human thermal comfort and respiratory health. Vapor pressure and moisture conditions of the air have a direct impact on both the thermal comfort and the respiratory health of humans. While long-standing comfort zones identify an acceptable relative humidity range of 20%–80%, more recent studies indicate that a much narrower range (between 40% and 60%) is necessary to maintain healthy respiratory conditions (Taylor & Hugentobler, 2016). In addition, emerging research about the appropriate humidity levels for maintaining a healthy indoor microbiome, while also alleviating pathogen propagation and residence times, is being developed (Leung et al., 2019). Humidity sensors allow for real-time localized data collection and provide unique insights on the concomitant relations between moisture levels and PM when combined with air quality sensing.

Most of our buildings incorporate potable water systems, as well as wastewater systems, for human health functions. The quality of our potable water is often challenged through the factors of plumbing materials, treatment methods, residence times, and flow rates. In some cases, waterborne illnesses are vast and have long-term effects on human health, such as lead poisoning in urban populations as exemplified in Detroit and similar communities (Pauli, 2020). Sensing techniques already exist to ensure that the potable water is safe for drinking and human consumption, but such technologies are not widely distributed or accessible due to affordability. Most US water utilities do not take responsibility for premise plumbing systems, which transition at the property line between municipal mains and into buildings. Building reentry practices and future occupancy reductions due to pandemic situations will have a large impact on water quality through both longer residence times and reduced flow rates relative to premise plumbing sizing. Sensing technologies for assessing this realm of building science and human health is becoming more important to reinform plumbing system materials and design for future adaptations. Wastewater systems are also indicators of human health based on biochemical analysis of wastewater sampling. Sampling techniques have become highly useful as early indicators of the useful for SARS-CoV-2 tracing, providing insight into infection sources as much as ten days in advance of symptomatic conditions experienced by humans (Betancourt et al., 2021). Such sensing techniques allow for early detection, tracing, and spread prevention for disease outbreaks.

Participatory Sensing

An online survey platform (e.g., Qualtrics) has expanded accessibility due to its internet connection and has streamlined data analytics of collected data. In other words, once a person possesses any connected device, they can readily share their perceptions. Benefiting from this potential, a new concept of participatory sensing emerged: users of such a platform actively participate in creating information using their human capabilities. For example, a navigation app, called Waze, allows users to report the location of police officers and/or any obstacles on a road. It supports a large-scale study that evaluates, for example, a building-level thermal comfort; hence, Huizenga et al. (2006) reported that only 11% of buildings out of 215 fulfilled the criterion of satisfying 80% of occupants – an underwhelming performance. Another route that takes advantage of is to collect a sufficient number of individual data, which paves the way for personal models. Daum et al. (2011) pioneered to develop a personalized measure of thermal comfort using 6,851 data from 28 human subjects. Often, a 5- or 7-point Likert scale is used to gather each user's perceptions (e.g., cold, cool, slightly cool, neutral, slightly warm, warm, hot) along with environmental data. Then, it becomes a pipeline for building systems (e.g., HVAC or lighting) to better serve occupants.

Human Biosensing

A biosensor is a device which utilizes a biological recognition system that transforms information about a specific analyte (a chemical substance being analyzed) concentration in a sample and, through a transducer, transforms the measurement into a quantifiable signal which is useful for data analysis purposes (Thevenot et al., 2001). A characteristic of human biosensing is that the biological measurement obtained by the recognition system is highly specific for the specific analyte or substrate being quantified. Without this specificity for either an analyte or a group of cells, for example, the oxygenation of blood, human biosensing would not be a viable or valuable tool (Thevenot et al., 2001). It was in Cincinnati, Ohio, in the 1950s that Leland C. Clark, Jr., became the father of biosensors, creating a biosensor for just that, determining the oxygen level in blood. After the failure of his first sensor, which could not separate blood components from the surface of the electrode receptor or recognition system, he used a cellophane wrapper from a cigarette pack to reduce the current. This allowed for only substances like oxygen, with a low molecular weight, to be measured. This model is still replicated successfully today, and Teflon is used in a Clark electrode (Renneberg et al., 2008). A human biosensor turns the level of an analyte in the individual to a quantifiable and applicable number through transduction; this is one of its main features. Due to the specificity and wide range of human biosensors available, there are several different ways an analyte can be measured to better understand a human's health condition. For example, cortisol is a known hormone released as a response to stress in humans. Having elevated cortisol over time is linked to a host of negative health conditions, such as prolonged wound healing or increased rate of cancer growth (Runyon et al., 2019). In a study aimed to observe the way cortisol behaves and metabolizes in humans, Runyon et al. (2019) collected human sweat in a laboratory setting during exercise using a pump adapted with a cold trap to collect human sweat directly, via vacuum, to the sample test tube. These samples were stored at very low temperatures until they were thawed for biosensing to detect the levels of cortisol in the sweat obtained (Runyon et al., 2019). This is just one example of the many analytes a biosensor could focus on measuring to gain a better understanding of what causes the analyte to elevate in an individual's body or to know what treatments to pursue after understanding more details obtained from the biosensor. This type of biosensor as well as other types, therefore, have many applications, a main feature of one of them being the ability to measure human stress and relaxation responses to a variety of environmental conditions.

Neurosensing

Neurosensing technologies that give us a deeper understanding of brain activity have the potential to expand our understanding of the relationship between neuroscience and built environments. An individual's brains activity is typically detected and recorded via electroencephalogram (EEG), a test which detects the electrical activity in the brain by using small electrodes attached to an individual's scalp. The brain's electrical activity shows up as wavy lines on an EEG display and recording. This occurs even when a person is asleep, since brain cells always stay active and communicate via electrical impulses (Mayo Clinic, n.d.).

Aspinall et al. (2015) in their study used a low-cost mobile EEG to assess the emotional impact of different urban environments and how urban green spaces could potentially reduce stress and frustration, and stimulate individuals at the same time. Exposure to different built environments has been known to shape adult cognitive functions. In this study, the EEG was used to record and analyze the emotional experience of a group of walkers in three different types of urban environments. This study exemplifies how neurosensing technologies can give researchers a deeper understanding of how the human brain reacts to the surrounding built environment. The findings have the potential to create physical environments conducive to human health and wellbeing. In this particular case, researchers used the EEG as a sensing mechanism to recognize human emotions and support urban green space as a mood-enhancing environment for all forms of physical activity (Aspinall et al., 2015).

Neuroscience research and neurosensing technologies, until the recent years, have been typically constrained to cables that connect to a computer for recording and analysis. Researchers at Brown University, however, developed a wireless brain sensing system that had the ability to acquire neural data during animal behavior experiments in 2014. This wireless neurosensor could record the full spectrum of electrophysiological signals from the cortex of nonhuman primates during sleep-wake transitions (Yin et al., 2014). These findings opened various opportunities for untethered neurological research. A neurosensor that does not rely on constrained communication could now allow individuals to move around in different types of indoor, outdoor, or transitional spaces, leading to findings which may positively impact the field of health and the built environment.

Chen et al. (2015) used a wireless EEG headset to measure brain waves in terms of amplitude. Participants in this study were asked to sit in either a natural environment or a built environment for 20 minutes, while the EEG was used to measure brain waves and function during the exposure. Researchers found that the large-amplitude synchronized EEG waves were expressed in the natural environment. They indicated that a natural environment may promote better brain performance (Chen et al., 2015). This study also demonstrated how untethered neurosensing technology could help further exploration into human health and wellbeing in different types of environments. Further, wireless neurosensors and other emerging technology in neurosensing could expand the fundamental understanding of the meaning of brainwaves.

Material Sensing

All materials are comprised of molecular structures that determine the material's properties. There are a range of characteristics that can be established for materials based on using sensors and other instruments to collect material-scale data. For the purpose of this book, material properties that have an impact on human health will be addressed. Some of the basic material sensing variables of interest include thermal properties, optical properties, and sorption and diffusion properties. Both the chemistry and molecular bonding patterns, as well as the fabrication process, define a material's characteristics. In addition, there is a distinction of the sensing tools that are used for collecting material data in the field as opposed to collecting data from materials in laboratories. The mobile, or *in situ*, sensing tools are primarily referenced in this book because of their significance for correlating field test data alongside human biosensing and environmental sensing measures.

Microbial Sensing

The ability to sense relatively invisible matter, such as microbes, particulates, and pathogens, is beneficial to determine potential human health impacts of a given environmental condition. Microbial sensing can take place in different media, such as air, water, or materials, and may be conducted *in situ* or through samples collected from a site that are then tested in a lab. The mobile sensing capabilities for microscale phenomena are rapidly expanding, especially with recent societal challenges such as the COVID-19 pandemic and the need for sensing nanoscale bioparticles that may be harmful to human respiratory systems.

Microbe sensing of air, water, and materials is becoming of greater and greater interest as the world of microbes and pathogens seems to be ever-expanding. Different measures are collected for microbial presence, whether characterization of microbe size, concentration, or other. Most *in situ* microbial sensors function through electrical transduction principles, while some laboratory sensing techniques function through optical, pH, and other biochemistry measures (Stieve, 1983).

Data Acquisition

There are different modes by which data can be collected and organized from sensing tools. The modes should be determined primarily based on the end-use goal or need for the data. Oftentimes, parsing and filtering of datasets are required prior to its usefulness in identifying informative results. The time interval of data collection is also predetermined based on the length, needs, and level of resolution for the study. Prior to acquiring data through sensors, it is best to establish the intended use and outcomes, unless the study is purely experimental and not driven by a hypothesis. Furthermore, when collecting multiple data types for a comparative analysis, it is best to align the situational contexts (i.e., time and location) of data acquisition. For instance, one would not want to collect environmental data from a site during a week in February and then collect human biosensing data from the same site during a week in August and make an attempt to use the results together for analysis. So, when moving towards a rigorous research or practice of data collection with multiple variables, the acquisition intervals, location, and timeframe should align as close as possible.

The placement of sensors for data acquisition is also a significant consideration, especially when dealing with varied environmental conditions in a given indoor or outdoor environment. Human biosensing technology placement is more obvious, with appropriate locations being predetermined by the sensing technique (i.e., wrist-devices, scalp EEG sensors, etc.). Knowledge about the general spatial environment, thermodynamics, human occupancy patterns, and the phenomena at hand will be necessary before determining the appropriate sensor locations for good-quality data acquisition. Some basic rules of thumb for setting up different sensing collection scenarios are identified in Chapter 2.3.

Environmental Data

There are numerous aspects of the environment that are of interest for both building functions and human health. Data can be collected for indoor and outdoor air quality, potable water, wastewater, heat, light, humidity, sound, and vibrational noise. Climate data informs the characterization of outdoor environmental conditions, including temperature, radiation, light, atmospheric refraction indices, cloud cover versus clear-sky conditions, relative humidity rainfall and precipitation, wind speed and direction and frequency, and refined variations of these aspects (i.e., direct normal, direct horizontal, and global radiation). Typical meteorological year (TMY) climate data is collated from a 30-year history of hourly datasets and statistically analyzed to provide a typical year of 8,760 data points for each phenomenon (Ebrahimpour & Maerefat, 2010). Indoor environmental data can be collected with different sensors, either commercially available or constructed from sensor kits (i.e., Arduino, Photon, etc.). The data collection for indoor environmental data can be calibrated to different resolutions depending on the study or ongoing monitoring requirements. We can utilize environmental data from both outdoor and indoor conditions to characterize the physiochemical, thermodynamic, and other conditions that may be impacting human functions and wellbeing. As sensing data collected from the environment is spatially specific, it is necessary to identify the spatial conditions alongside data collection zones. For example, climate data is typically collected from weather stations that are located at regional airports at 10 meters above the ground. If we are interested in the microclimate conditions surrounding a specific building or urban space, it is best to consider placing a local weather station at the area of interest since many factors influence the climate data (urban form creating shading masks and airflow modifications, bodies of water or parks creating humidity and temperature differences, etc.) (Lembrechts et al., 2021).

Human Perception Data

As a way of reflecting individual's perception quantitatively, surveys are often implemented. In the past, distributing surveys (e.g., paper-based questionnaires) was a time-consuming and costly solution; therefore, it was performed sporadically without any specific guidelines. However, as noted, the internet capability and online platforms for survey development (e.g., Qualtrics) streamlined collecting human perception data and led to a paradigm shift in operating building systems like HVAC and lighting (e.g., personalization).

There is also a movement of creating a large-scale dataset as human perception data, especially with contextual and environmental data (e.g., the building type, HVAC type, air temperature, etc.) For example, the ASHRAE Global Thermal Comfort Database II (Ličina et al., 2018) contained approximately 81,846 complete sets of indoor environmental and subjective evaluation data. Given that the proliferation of data-driven methods like machine/deep learning affects every field and the number of quality data plays a significant role, researchers are gathered together to facilitate developments in the field, especially where human perceptions are the determinants.

Human Productivity and Performance Data

The relationship between human productivity/performance and indoor environments has been examined over decades. In the modern era, where people conduct a variety of works indoors, the complexity of measuring human productivity/performance increased. The transition from manufacturing-based to knowledge-based work among office workers is an example. Researchers started exploring different ways to collect such data. For example, in recent years, self-reported assessment surveys are used more frequently (e.g., Gupta et al., 2020) despite their subjectiveness. Cognitive performance tests have been employed consistently in the studies to quantify office worker performance indirectly. The objectiveness, readily acquired by performing these tests, could have attracted researchers. Moreover, these tests allow more control in the experiments' design since participants would conduct the same work. Under the conceptualization that behavior is impacted by cognition, emotion, and executive functions, the studies wanted to relate the cognitive and information-processing components to office work performance. Quantitative studies in offices such as call center staff's performance (Fisk et al.,

2002) or the number of files processed by workers (Kroner, 1994) became more common.

Human Bioresponse Data

Human biosensing devices collect biological measurements which are highly specific for the analyte or substrate that is being quantified. Researchers can collect human bioresponsive data in a variety of ways. Runyon et al. (2019) measured and studied sweat as a noninvasive measurement tool for biomarkers. These researchers, by analyzing sweat, identified a variety of biomarkers that correlated with stress, fatigue, hydration, cancer, cognition, appetite, and nutrition. Sweat samples for this study were collected from four healthy volunteers for whom sweat was induced via exercise on a stationary bike and was then collected using a portable handheld battery-operated pump. This data has useful potential for making associations between human health, physical activity, and environmental conditions.

This team, along with other researchers at the University of Arizona, is now working on hands-free collection devices to deliver standardized and high-quality sweat samples which can be tested for biomarkers. The ultimate goal is to develop noninvasive wearable devices to detect sweat biomarkers, which can monitor individual health continuously and in real time, and do not require the collection of blood (UAHS, 2020).

Neurological Data

Neurological data in the field of health and the built environment is typically acquired by analyzing brainwaves and determining what they mean in the context of the environment. For example, in the previously discussed study by Aspinall et al. (2015), researchers used an EEG that involved 14 sensors that were positioned on the participant's scalp. They measured the brainwaves in terms of amplitude and frequency and further indicated that the four main independent bands are δ (0.5–4 Hz), which shows deep sleep, and conversely excitement or agitation when delta waves are suppressed; θ (4–8 Hz), which expresses deep meditative states and automatic tasks; α (8–15 Hz), indicating alertness and restful and meditative states; and β (15–30 Hz), indicating wakefulness, mental engagement, and conscious processing of information. Aspinall et al. (2015) then performed a high-dimensional correlated component regression analysis of these brainwaves to determine the results of their experiment. These researchers thereby demonstrated that brainwaves, which are electrical impulses in the brain, can indicate a variety of things about an individual's behavior and emotion. This also reveals how research involving neurological measures and data has significant potential to make an impact on human health and wellbeing via its relationship with built environments.

Material Data

Material data comes in a variety of forms – it might ascribe qualitative conditions of surface structure (i.e., rough, smooth) or quantitative values of density or porosity. Each measure tells us something about a material's characteristics for design. For instance, a rough surface structure will bounce light in a Lambertian distribution pattern resulting in diffuse reflection. While a smooth material surface will reflect light equal to the angle of incidence, resulting in specular reflection. High-density materials may be indicative of thermally conductive properties, while porous structures are more thermally resistant. Material data is often characterized through microscopy techniques such as scanning electron microscopy (SEM) imaging, which virtually separates layers or strata of a material by electron signals to collect spatial information, then rebuilds the layers into a composite image. SEM images are useful in providing structural properties and specific measures of material structure (i.e., length of polymer chain, size of pore, etc.). Interpretations of the images are made through scientific principles and observation.

Microbiome Data

Interest in the microbiome is growing rapidly as it is an area where thousands of different microbial species are being discovered and identified as helpful, potentially harmful to human health, or benign. Some microorganisms are beneficial and necessary for production of oxygen and nutrients for plants, decomposing organic materials, and maintaining certain aspects of human health (i.e., probiotics for the gut microbiome). However, others are pathogenic (viruses in particular) and can cause diseases in other living species (plants, animals, and humans). Datasets for microbes may be grouped by different types of microorganisms based on cellular composition (range): viruses (nanometer), archaea (0.5–4.0 microns), bacteria (0.5–5.0 microns), fungi (2–10 microns), protozoa (1–150 microns), and algae (5–1,000 microns).

The microbiome of outdoor and indoor spaces is uniquely different, primarily because of the soils, flora, and fauna that exist in the outdoors compared to controlled ventilation and somewhat sanitized indoor environments. Of course, there is a spectrum of differences in microbiomes, both outdoors and indoors, depending on the general composition of biological specimens that are present (i.e., a dog park or a zoo will have a different set of microbes compared to a recreational ski slope, or a hospital may have more pathogens present compared to a typical office building). Studies being conducted at the University of Oregon's Biology and the Built Environment Center (BioBe) are engaging specifically with deepening our understanding of the microbiome towards improving human health and environmental sustainability (BioBe, 2023).

ROI Data

The built environment industry designs and constructs the world's buildings, infrastructure, cities, and landscapes. It impacts the economy, the environment, and overall human health and wellbeing. It is critical, therefore, to identify a healthy built environment framework which includes research that examines the relationship between the built environment and human health (Berke & Vernez-Moudon, 2014). Building on knowledge which informs stakeholders' decisions in design and construction has the potential to have an enormous impact in the field of design and health.

When equipped with advanced sensing technologies and data acquisition, researchers, designers, and decision-makers can collaborate towards the creation of built environments that are catalysts for positive impact on human health. Research studies using these technologies and methods, however, come with many time and budget considerations. In order to implement research findings into the real world, therefore, a sound ROI model is required for administrators, developers, business owners, and other decision-makers.

Researchers need to assist their collaborators in the field in translating research findings to design outcomes for healthy environments. Figueiro (2008), for example, studied the influence of different lighting interventions on older adults and proposed a 24-hour lighting scheme to improve their visual environments and sleep efficiency. If this lighting proposal were to be implemented in a senior living community, we could, thereafter, conduct post-occupancy studies to generate actual ROI data which may demonstrate a positive health impact on occupants of that community. This is a good example of how ROI data can help businesses develop and better market senior living communities that promote health and wellness in older adults. All sensing and data acquisition tools and methods discussed in this chapter have the ability to provide this ROI data for different building types. Ultimately, this information has a significant impact on how buildings are designed and constructed.

References

American Society of Heating, Refrigerating, and Air-conditioning Engineers (ASHARE). (2019) Ventilation for acceptable indoor air quality. ASHRAE 62.1 Standard.

Aqilah, N., Rijal, H. B., & Zaki, S. A. (2022). A review of thermal comfort in residential buildings: Comfort threads and energy saving potential. *Energies, 15*(23), 9012. https://doi.org/10.3390/en15239012

ASHRAE. (2020). Thermal environmental conditions for human occupancy. ASHRAE 55 Standard.

Aspinall, P., Mavros, P., Coyne, R., & Roe, J. (2015). The urban brain: Analysing outdoor physical activity with mobile EEG. *British Journal of Sports Medicine, 49*(4), 272–276.

Berke, E. M., & Vernez-Moudon, A. (2014). Built environment change: A framework to support health-enhancing behaviour through environmental policy and health research. *Journal of Epidemiology Community Health, 68*(6), 586–590.

Betancourt, W. Q., Schmitz, B. W., Innes, G. K., Prasek, S. M., Pogreba Brown, K. M., Stark, E. R., Foster, A. R., Sprissler, R. S., Harris, D. T., Sherchan, S. P., Gerba, C. P., & Pepper, I. L. (2021). COVID-19 containment on a college campus via wastewater-based epidemiology, targeted clinical testing and an intervention. *The Science of the Total Environment, 779*, 146408–146408. https://doi.org/10.1016/j.scitotenv.2021.146408

BioBe (Biology and the Build Environment). (2023). University of Oregon. Retrieved from https://biobe.uoregon.edu/

Chen, Z., He, Y., & Yu, Y. (2015). Natural environment promotes deeper brain functional connectivity than built environment. *BMC Neuroscience, 16*(S1), 294.

Daum, D., Haldi, F., & Morel, N. (2011). A personalized measure of thermal comfort for building controls. *Building and Environment, 46*, 3–11.

DiLaura, D., Houser, K., Mistrick, R., & Steffy, G. (Eds.) (2014). *The lighting handbook*. New York: Illuminating Engineering Society of North America.

Ebrahimpour, A., & Maerefat, M. (2010). A method for generation of typical meteorological year. *Energy Conversion and Management, 51*(3), 410–417.

Figueiro, M. G. (2008). A proposed 24 hour lighting scheme for older adults. *Lighting Research & Technology, 40*(2), 153–160.

Fisk, W. J., Price, P., Faulkner, D., Sullivan, D., Dibartolomeo, D., Federspiel, C., Liu, G. & Lahiff, M. (2002). Worker Productivity and Ventilation Rate in a Call Center: Analyses of Time-Series Data for a Group of Workers. Indoor Air 2002, 1, 1–20. https://escholarship.org/uc/item/55d3h8zd

Gupta, R., Howard, A., & Zahiri, S. (2020). Defining the link between indoor environment and workplace productivity in a modern UK office building. *Architectural Science Review, 63*(3–4), 248–261.

Huizenga, C., Abbaszadeh, S., Zagreus, L. and Arens, E. (2006). Air Quality and Thermal Comfort in Office Buildings: Results of a Large Indoor Environmental Quality Survey. Proceedings of Healthy Buildings, 3, 393–397.

Irwin, R. J., & Corballis, M. C. (1968). On the general form of Stevens' law for loudness and softness. *Perception & Psychophysics, 3*, 137–143. https://doi.org/10.3758/BF03212781

Kroner, W. M. (1994). Environmentally responsive workstations and office-worker productivity. *ASHRAE Transactions, 100*(2), 750–755.

LeGates, T. A., Fernandez, D. C., & Hattar, S. (2014). Light as a central modulator of circadian rhythms, sleep and affect. *Nature Reviews Neuroscience, 15*(7), 443–454.

Lembrechts, Lenoir, J., Scheffers, B., De Frenne, P., & Algar, A. (2021). Designing countrywide and regional microclimate networks. *Global Ecology and Biogeography, 30*(6), 1168–1174. https://doi.org/10.1111/geb.13290

Leung, Marcus. H. Y., Tong, Xinzhao., & Lee, Patrick. K. H. (2019). Indoor microbiome and airborne pathogens. *Comprehensive Biotechnology*, (6)96–106. Indoor Microbiome and Airborne Pathogens Leung, Marcus HY; Tong, Xinzhao; Lee, Patrick KH. ISBN: 9780444640468; DOI: 10.1016/B978-0-444-64046-8.00477-8 Comprehensive Biotechnology, 2019, Vol.6, p.96–106 https://doi.org/10.1016/B978-0-444-64046-8.00477-8 ISBN: 9780444640468

Ličina, V. F., Cheung, T., & Zhang, H., et al. (2018). Development of the ASHRAE Global thermal comfort Database II. *Building and Environment, 142*, 502–512.

Mayo Clinic. (n.d.). *EEG (electroencephalogram)*. Retrieved March 26, 2020 from https://www.mayoclinic.org/tests-procedures/eeg/about/pac-20393875

Mikulka, M. (2018, June 19). The ultimate guide to light measurement [Blog post]. Retrieved from https://www.lumitex.com/blog/light-measurement#1

Pauli, B. J. (2020). The Flint water crisis. *WIREs Water, 7*, e1420. https://doi.org/10.1002/wat2.1420

Prüss-stün, A., & Corvalán, C. (2006). What is the environment in the context of health? In *Preventing disease through healthy environments: Towards an estimate of the environmental burden of disease* (pp. 20–23). Geneva, Switzerland: World Health Organization. https://www.who.int/publications/i/item/9241593822. ISBN: 9241593822, 11 June 2006, Global report

Renneberg, R., Pfeiffer, D., Lisdat, F. Wilson, G., Wollenberger, U., Ligler, F., & Turner, A. P. F. (2008). Frieder Scheller and the short history of biosensors. In R. Renneberg & F. Lisdat (Eds.), *Biosensing for the 21st century* (pp. 1–18). Berlin, Heidelberg: Springer.

Runyon, J. R., Jia, M., Goldstein, M. R., Skeath, P., Abrell, L., Chorover, J., & Sternberg, E. M. (2019). Dynamic behavior of cortisol and cortisol metabolites in human eccrine sweat. *International Journal of Prognostics and Health Management, 10*, 1–11.

Seppänen, O. A., Fisk, W. J., & Mendell, M. J. (1999). Association of ventilation rates and CO2 concentrations with health and other responses in commercial and institutional buildings. *Indoor Air, 9*(4), 226–252

Stieve, Hennig. (1983). Sensors of biological organisms — biological transducers. *Sensors and Actuators, 4*, 689–704.

Taylor, S., & Hugentobler, W. (2016). Is low indoor humidity a driver for healthcare-associated infections? In *Indoor Air 2016*. Belgium. Published: Nov 2016 | Poster session, "INDOOR AIR 2016" Conference in Ghent, Belgium. https://www.condairgroup.com/humidity-health-wellbeing/scientific-studies/is-low-indoor-humidity-a-driver-for-healthcare-associated-infections

Thevenot, D. R., Toth, K., Durst, R. A., & Wilson, G. S. (2001). Electrochemical biosensors: Recommended definitions and classifications. *Analytical Letters, 34*(5), 635–659.

United States Environmental Protection Agency [USEPA]. (2016a, December 20). NAAQS table. Retrieved from https://www.epa.gov/criteria-air-pollutants/naaqs-table

United States Environmental Protection Agency [USEPA]. (2016b, October 18). Table of historical lead (Pb) national ambient air quality standards (NAAQS). Retrieved from https://www.epa.gov/lead-air-pollution/table-historical-lead-pb-national-ambient-air-quality-standards-naaqs

United States Environmental Protection Agency [USEPA]. (2019, July 3). Managing air quality: Air pollutant types. Retrieved from https://www.epa.gov/air-quality-management- process/managing-air-quality-air-pollutant-types

University of Arizona Health Sciences (UAHS). (2020, February 13). Scientists study sweat, the small stuff. Retrieved from https://uahs.arizona.edu/news/scientists-study-sweat-small-stuff

Yin, M., Borton, D. A., Komar, J., Agha, N., Lu, Y., Li, H., ... & Larson, L. (2014). Wireless neurosensor for full-spectrum electrophysiology recordings during free behavior. *Neuron, 84*(6), 1170–1182.

5 Measurement Tools and Technologies

Introduction

The tools and technologies that are necessary for the sensing data collection aspects of human, environment, and material measures are discussed in this chapter. Current state-of-the-art noninvasive, wearable biosensor devices alongside embedded material sensors and environmental sensor packages now give us the means to quantify stress, health, and wellness outcomes in different built environments. Expanded measurement technologies include neurosensing to inform the brain science of built environment impact and microbial sensing to help characterize the microbiome. Tools used for other aspects of human health and wellbeing research for built environments are discussed. These include virtual reality (VR) headsets, life cycle analysis (LCA) calculation tools, fisheye lens photography tools, and machine/deep learning algorithms. Each of these tools and technologies is enabling new ways of considering the impacts of built environment design on human health and wellbeing. These technologies are ever-changing in a rapidly advancing field, so the general necessity for considering appropriate modes of measurement (sensing, simulation, calculation, survey, photograph, etc.) is discussed. Additionally, this chapter addresses the fundamental science and knowledge for how these sensing technologies and measurement tools function in application.

Sensing Technologies

A variety of emerging and advanced technologies, including environmental sensors, noninvasive biosensors, and neurosensors that can quantify stress and other biomarkers of individual health and wellbeing within the built environment, are discussed below (Figure 5.1).

DOI: 10.4324/9780367814748-8

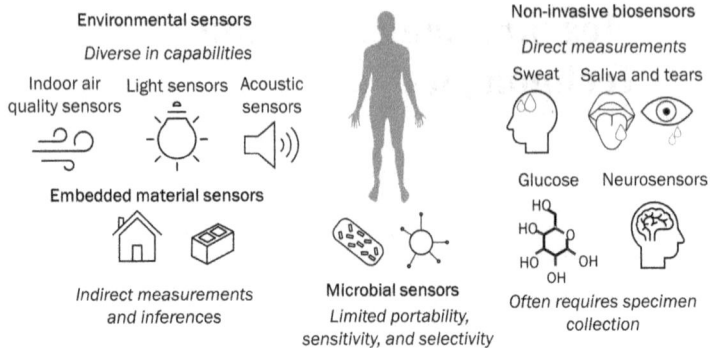

Figure 5.1 Composite Diagram: Comparative Diagrams of Various Sensing Devices and Technologies.

Environmental Sensors

Environmental sensors are diverse in their capabilities which include measurements of pollutants and toxins in water, soil, and air – indoor as well as outdoor – and levels of light, sound, gases, temperature, and humidity. All these features are immensely useful for employers and individuals to assess how these levels of different environmental elements influence health and wellbeing.

Monitoring, analyzing, and understanding air quality data and integrating it into policy used to reside only with of the US Environmental Protection Agency (U.S. EPA) but now environmental air quality sensors are commercially available to the public. Individuals with access can view their results remotely or in person. These sensors can now monitor and measure ambient indoor and outdoor data, in real time and continuously (Aeroqual, 2019). These products are very valuable in creating a basic understanding of different types of pollutants in a particular space, area, or region, and where and how interventions need to be made to mitigate these pollutants. Today's generation, which spends more time indoors than ever before, however, faces unique challenges. Globally, it is estimated that approximately 90% of an individual's time is spent indoors (Challoner et al., 2015). This estimate, however, may vary based on geography and culture. For example, while 25% of Americans surveyed in one study spent over 20 hours per day indoors, European countries tend to be on a more conservative scale with 38% of survey respondents reporting being indoors for 15–20 hours per day (Licea, 2018). It is important to consider how much time individuals are spending indoors because indoor air quality (IAQ) is oftentimes worse than outdoor air quality, a phenomenon which is perpetuated by lack of IAQ monitoring and regulations (Challoner et al., 2015).

IAQ Sensors

A majority of IAQ studies have focused on health, productivity, and performance in work settings. Their findings reveal decreased productivity due to sinus irritation, headaches, and other ailments related to poor IAQ (Challoner et al., 2015). Studies of this nature have now made IAQ monitors popular and marketable for research as well as everyday use. Most IAQ monitors track a combination of all or any of a number of IAQ indicators including but not limited to temperature, humidity, volatile organic compounds (VOCs), particulate matter (PM), carbon dioxide (CO_2), ozone, and other gases. Along with these features, some are even more multifunctional; they can mechanically filter air on a schedule with a fan or other type of appliance to mitigate a pollutant or stagnant air (Ansaldo, 2019).

Examples of the types of IAQ measuring sensors available to individuals, businesses, institutions, or agencies are the Google Nest Protect, designed more to be used by individuals or families, and Sensirion's environmental sensors, aimed more at organizations that want to track IAQ. The Google Nest Protect is more than just a smoke alarm; while it measures both fast burning and smoldering fires, it also functions as a carbon monoxide detector that tests itself every month and lasts over ten years. It also functions as a night light in a hallway, and it has software intelligent enough to differentiate between steam and smoke in a house, thereby reducing the number of times one would need to silence it, an action which can be performed from one's phone (Google, n.d.). Since it is connected wirelessly to personal phones, in the event of an overexposure to carbon monoxide or smoke, individuals could be alerted even when they are away from home. For corporate and organization use, Sensirion's environmental sensors may be more applicable. They measure CO_2, VOCs, $PM_{2.5}$ and PM_{10}, relative humidity (RH), and temperature (T). One sensor does not measure all of these, however, as the sensors are uniquely outfitted to the individual task or need. For example, one sensor marketed by Sensirion is the CO_2 & RH/T Sensor Module, meant for applications in HVAC systems and IAQ measurements. This sensor is not only equipped with precise CO_2, humidity, and temperature monitors with the goal of improving health and quality of the indoor environment, but also to be energy efficienct (Sensirion, 2020).

Light Sensors

Environmental light sensors measure the quality and quantity of light in an environment to provide valuable data to potentially find associations with occupants' performance, productivity, circadian rhythms, sense of wellbeing, mood, and other indicators of health. The World Health Organization (WHO) recommends 5–15 minutes of sunlight exposure two to three times per week, based on the necessary amount of natural radiation exposure to aid in the production of vitamin D ("UV Radiation", 2019). Previous research studies, however, have found long-standing associations between improvements in light quality in built environments and improvements in productivity and health individually as well as collectively. One pilot study performed by Konis and colleagues in a dementia care setting suggests that exposure to daylight for two hours daily reduces depression severity on a special scale meant for dementia patients, compared to those who did not have the presence of natural light in their built environments (2018). Light sensors, therefore, are particularly applicable and important in institutional settings for special populations whose circadian rhythms can be disrupted due to low levels of light (Konis et al., 2018).

Environmental light sensors such as luxmeters have the ability to measure light levels in almost any environment, measuring illuminance in lux (lx) or foot-candles (fc). These meters can measure high natural lighting levels which may reach approximately 100,000 lx or electric lighting levels in workspaces which tend to be at around 500 lx on average (IWBI, 2017). Computer simulations in different types of available software are also able to show the distribution of illuminance throughout a room in specific weather conditions, such as cloudy or sunny. These computer renderings look similar to a heat map and have their light measurements in lux above the clusters of different light intensities (Velux, n.d.).

Proving both the physiological and psychological benefits of natural light can be complex, and environmental light sensors can play a significant role in this regard. Zadeh et al. (2014) studied nurses in a workplace setting with or without windows in different parts of the same hospital using physiological assessments such as blood pressure, level of oxygen saturation, and body temperature alongside behavioral assessments, such as measuring levels of alertness or medication errors. They also used digital light meters to measure illumination levels. Although the results were not statistically significant, they found a 22% decrease in medication errors in the group which had a window in their work area and higher natural light illumination levels (Zadeh et al., 2014). This study reveals the usefulness of environmental digital light meters; they were important to show that one group was exposed to more sunlight.

Acoustic Sensors

Environmental sensors used to measure the acoustics in different built environments can similarly be correlated with other measures of wellbeing to reveal significant results in research studies. Although most measures of noise pollution tend to be brief, they can provide a great amount of insight into the potential damage on individual health and mitigation strategies that can be employed if sound is also captured with geographic information. Data from noise maps can be helpful in determining how the built environment can be designed to identify and reduce problems with acoustics. There are several types of environmental sensors which measure acoustics and noise, ranging from a smartphone with apps to specific ear simulation transducers. Manufacturers usually provide compatible software, which are specific to the intended use and outcomes (Wessels & Basten, 2016).

Noninvasive Biosensors

Noninvasive biosensors, one of the cutting-edge technological advances within the 21st century, are chemical sensors that recognize components based on biological or biochemical mechanisms of the human body (Banica, 2012). The challenge with noninvasive biosensors, however, is avoiding the need to physically draw the blood to determine the level of a biological component within the body. For example, an invasive biosensor would be the typical method of measurement for blood glucose in a diabetic patient by using a biosensor which reads the level of an enzyme in the blood by directly drawing the blood. There are many noninvasive biosensors currently being tested for the efficiency, reliability, and accuracy, which may soon be used as mainstream practice. One example of this is the GlucoWatch which was first studied and developed in 2001 (Tierney et al., 2001). This device attempted to use a technique called reverse iontophoresis, which is a transdermal application of noninvasive biosensors. Iontophoresis is a process which uses electrical fields to attract molecules of interest, or analytes, from the dermal layer of the skin containing blood vessels, through the most external layer of the skin, the epidermis, to the sensor which emits a signal based on the levels of the targeted analyte (Giri et al., 2017). A clinical evaluation of this method was performed in 2001, which showed that not only was it efficient, but it was as accurate as the method it was compared to drawing the blood via finger-pricking (Tierney et al., 2001). Since less than 3% of cases showed skin irritation, it leads to some questions about why it was removed from the market in 2007. Some limitations of this method were that resistance of dry human skin varies widely which requires careful calibration (Giri et al., 2017). Many other types of noninvasive biosensors exist, such as saliva-, tear-, and sweat-based biosensors. Saliva, tears, and sweat are all valuable biofluids because they each have unique analytes which can be studied and transduced from chemical information to a display which can be used as a diagnostic tool. For example, uric acid is an analyte found in sweat, whereas fluoride is an analyte found in saliva (Bandodkar & Wang, 2014). However, there are some analytes which are common and found in all these biofluids. While it is helpful to collect and use biofluid samples similar to the way the blood is drawn and analyzed, some biosensors for saliva sampling were developed for more permanence including placement inside of dentures or mouth guards (Bandodkar & Wang, 2014). While saliva is potentially useful to study in a lab even without biosensors, tears are extremely difficult to transport to a laboratory and assess without the use of a biosensor. Some tear-based biosensors are essentially flexible contact lenses with wireless electronics built in and are currently still in development phases for use. Real-world applications are not easily demonstrated, as particular care must be taken with the eye area (Bandodkar & Wang, 2014). One of the biggest challenges to overcome so far has been charging these devices. Sweat-based sensors contain physiological data, and many analytes in sweat are directly indicative of an individual's current health status. Human sweat contains thousands of potential analytes or biomarkers, ranging from proteins to small molecules or electrolyte components. These sensors are most commonly plastic-based, combined with other components as a temporary tattoo, or more like a skin patch or adhesive bandage (Runyon et al., 2019). Since the presence or quantity of specific biomarkers in sweat has been linked to the human health condition, specifically to stress, hydration, and cancer, the development of efficient sweat-based sensors is paramount. Currently under development for use are nonpermanent tattoos – noninvasive biosensors with the capability of giving researchers data about the specific analytes or biomarkers in an individual's sweat. One of the types of nonpermanent tattoos specifically measures pH and lactate when sweat interacts with the polymers in the tattoo that are sensitive to target analytes and cause a reaction. This specific tattoo is useful because the levels of lactate in an individual's sweat directly correlate to the amount of physical activity, which when tracked over time could show an individual's changes in stamina and performance during weight loss (UC San Diego, 2013).

Neurosensors

Neurosensors are considered to be expanded measurement technologies, but their historical use has been constrained because the sensors attached to the brain must be connected to a computer to analyze important electrical signals. These investigations have expanded the field of neuroscience and allowed a deeper understanding of human brain function. While evaluating electrical signals from the brain is undeniably critical for neuroscience research, relying on a tethered connection is a significant limitation that requires improvement. For example, a study performed by Yin et al. (2014) overcame this limitation by engineering a wireless neurosensor that was fully capable of recording the full range of electrophysiological brain signals. The study evaluated this wireless design by monitoring the sleep-wake transitions of nonhuman primates. The findings of this research revealed the safety of this neurosensor and its ability to perform neuroscience research in previously inaccessible locations (Yin et al., 2014). By demonstrating how wireless sensors can be safe and effective, this research also overcame the limitations of previous models of neurosensors. Capogrosso et al. (2016), in another study, developed a wireless control system that linked neural decoding of the extremities to bypass spinal cord injuries and promote walking movement in nonhuman primates. This study was similar to the one performed by Yin et al. (2014) because it allowed wireless analysis of the brain and spinal cord function. This advanced neurotechnology utilized wireless control systems to integrate the brain-spine interface. Once again, nontethered neurosensors are important for the advancement of neuroscience research because they allow studies of the brain that are not confined to a single space (Capogrosso et al., 2016). Brain activity can be indicative of an associated mood when encountering the built environment. Different environments can have different effects on the human brain which allows researchers to determine the stimuli that impact quality of life, psycho-emotional health, and overall health and wellbeing (Norwood et al., 2019). Further, different elements of the built environment can affect mood, sleep quality, and depressive systems. For these reasons, measuring the brain activity can assess the physiological impact of built environments (Norwood et al., 2019). There are now a variety of different neuroimaging techniques from the electroencephalography (EEG) to the functional magnetic resonance imaging (fMRI) that interpret the brain activity (Norwood et al., 2019). Findings from using advanced forms of neuroimaging techniques, including advanced techniques from researchers who did not need to tether patients to a computer, can positively influence how the built environment impacts human health and wellbeing.

Embedded Material Sensors

Obtaining material temperature data is useful for research and design of spaces for human thermal comfort, especially to inform the mean radiant temperature (MRT) that is factored into the thermal comfort equation. Localized material surface temperature sensors can be embedded within the material or in contact with the surface of the material, such as thermistors or contact temperature sensors. These sensor types, which function based on a thermocouple resistance differential, allow for the calibration to ambient temperatures and the customization of data intervals of interest. Ultimately, the thermistor data can depict intriguing thermal behaviors of materials in correlation with the surrounding air temperatures and radiant conditions (i.e., rapid or slow temperature change). Thermal imaging, or infrared (IR), cameras can also be used to assess the material temperatures of a given environment. The IR cameras are useful for visualizing the differences between various materials and their context as well as providing quick reference of bright spots (hot material temperatures) and dark spots (cold material temperatures). Thermal imaging is technically a process of collecting radiated IR wavelengths of light (780 nm–1 mm) emitting off of surfaces onto an internal sensor array, which then calculates the collected electromagnetic signals into a temperature value to create a color map (Lloyd, 2013). Other modes of light sensing for materials are also available and useful, especially to determine specific wavelengths occurring in the indoor environment that may be impacting or benefiting human health. Ultraviolet (UV) sensors will isolate the UV range (100–400 nm) into three specific bands: UVA (315–400 nm), UVB (280–315 nm), and UVC (100–280 nm). The separation of these bands of UV is significant as each band has proven to have different impacts on human health and other biological functions. UVC is the most damaging to biological functions, but generally, UVC is not reaching the earth being filtered out by atmospheric particles (though stratospheric ozone depletion is creating changes in UVC penetration). UV damage caused by UVC can lead to cell damage such as skin cancer, cataracts, and a weakened immune system (Ullrich, 2005), while UVB can cause skin aging and discoloration and potentially lead to skin cancer development. UVA is the least intrusive on biological functions and the most prevalent wavelength reaching the earth. UVA has proven useful for some technological advancements, such as photocatalysis when combined with oxidizing agents such as titanium dioxide (TiO_2), which provides indirect human health benefits such as air purification and water filtration processes. However, UVA also has direct human skin aging and darkening effects and can influence long-term development of skin cancer. Many building glazing technologies are designed to be spectrally selective and filter out UV light so that inhabitants can enjoy the benefits of natural light without the concern for UV exposure. UV sensors allow for the evaluation of existing built environments and provide data that can inform design improvements with new glazing materials or other light-control strategies. Visible (VIS) range light sensors are also available and can provide isolated bands for each color spectrum. As many designers are beginning to look more closely at the co-benefits of plants and living systems integrated within buildings and in the outdoor urban environment, the usefulness of VIS spectrum sensors allows us to determine the availability of specific wavelengths that are necessary for photosynthesis (blue and red wavelengths). Short wavelengths of VIS light also prove most beneficial for other biological functions, such as stabilizing and maintaining the human circadian rhythm, while long red wavelengths encourage relaxation and sleep (Sahin & Figueiro, 2013). Many studies on light and human biological functions prove the significance and importance of considering these values in the design of our building enclosures in particular because natural daylighting of interior spaces is dependent on the spatial organization of transmitting materials in relation to light accessible orientations. Incorporating light sensors in our environment helps researchers and designers understand the available spatiotemporal wavelengths for specific biological functions. Light transmission meters are often used for determining material transmittance values and can characterize the UV, VIS, and IR ranges. Photosensors, or photoelectric sensors, are the typical light sensing devices used in research activities as these can be basic and low cost as well as highly accurate and expensive, depending on project needs and resources. Photosensors can be placed on either side of a material to function similar to a light transmission meter and allow for real-time ongoing data collection, whereas most light transmission meters give a static readout based on the ambient source light at the time a material sample is tested. Water sensing is another area that is sometimes necessary for building material integration, especially for conditions that can lead to negative health impacts (i.e., mold and mildew). Some building materials are designed to be hydrophobic and reject moisture as well as minimize vapor transport (i.e., vapor barriers or retarders). Some materials, however, help to mediate ambient humidity levels, which can be beneficial for the human respiratory system, and incorporate advantageous sorption and/or diffusion processes. Most building materials, however, are negatively impacted when water infiltrates or interacts with the material chemistry, resulting in mold, mildew, calcification, rust, or patina. Integral hygrothermal sensors embedded in materials allow for real-time evaluation of moisture content levels. Building operators will sometimes incorporate hygrothermal sensors into the roofing materials or plumbing chase walls in order to detect leaks in critical facilities before the water source becomes problematic.

Microbial Sensors

Microbial sensing is based on developments from biochemical sensing and electrical transduction principles, which were pioneered in 1962 by Clark and Lyons (Clark, 1962). The biological interface will consist of an organism, tissue, cell, organelle, nucleic acid, enzyme, receptor, or antibody, while the transducer will be based on potentiometric, amperometric, conductimetric, impedimetric, calorimetric, optical, or acoustic properties (Mulchandani et al., 1998). The integrated transducer will generate a signal that indicates the level of analyte concentration within the biological specimen (Lim, 2015). The energy needed for transducer detection originates with the metabolism of the cell in the form of electrochemical gradients (Stieve, 1983). There are two main categories of conventional microbial sensors: optical detection methods (photon detectors, fluorescence microscopy, and chromatography techniques) and electrochemical detection methods (conductometric, amperometric, potentiometric, and voltammetric) (Lim, 2015). These conventional methods have some limitations, including limited portability, sensitivity, and selectivity. Other microbial sensing techniques are being developed with nanotechnological detection methods (microfluidic systems, microbioreactors, micro/nanofabrication, and micro/nanomaterials) (Lim, 2015). For the integration of microbial sensing with built environment spaces, portable methods are necessary, as are methods for integration with different medium types (airborne, waterborne, material-borne). Each medium in the built environment serves as a carrier and generator of potentially harmful pathogens or microbes that can affect human health. More rapid sensing and detection methods that are easily integrated with human-occupied indoor spaces will be helpful for real-time environmental health information. For research purposes, other modes for detecting microbes and pathogens can be employed by collecting sample from air, water, or materials on-site and then analyzing those specimens in an off-site laboratory.

Measurement Tools VR Headsets

A VR headset is a device that mounts on the wearer's head and provides an immersive and virtual experience for the user. While VR has gained widespread attention for its use in video games, it can also be used in a variety of other fields. For example, there is potential for VR to engage viewers in the visualization of buildings and infrastructures (Nikolić et al., 2019). VR can have positive impacts on human health by simulating healing environments that are safe, interactive, and easily duplicated (Rizzo, 2003). The built environment can have substantial impacts on human health and wellbeing, and VR can be an effective measurement tool related to this phenomenon. VR has become an effective technology that enables researchers to consider the impacts of the built environment's design and the affect that has on human health and wellbeing before it is actually constructed in the real world. The primary appeal of using VR in the predesign stage is its ability to produce elements of the built environment in a dynamic and compelling manner. For example, users can be immersed in a virtual environment where they can readily and accessibly navigate between different viewpoints and perspectives, permitting them to interact with an immersive environment in real time (Nikolić et al., 2019). Since VR provides an immersive physical environment, interactive measurement tools and methods related to health and wellbeing research are important to consider. Being immersively present in the VR environments allows users to examine different virtual objects and their dimensional properties. Measurements within the VR environment can allow the researcher to use sound judgment and perform manual measurements without having to construct the actual environment (Hagedorn et al., 2007). VR is, therefore, an important measurement tool because it can eliminate the confusion designers may have during the early conceptualization of designing buildings as well as help them anticipate problems and address user needs from the beginning.

LCA Calculation Tools

LCA refers to the quantitative and qualitative study and accounting of material sourcing, manufacturing and production, transport, implementation for intended use, operation and maintenance, and end-of-life or next-use purposing.

At each stage of the material's life, there is a series of metrics such as carbon emissions, energy consumption, and water consumption that are accounted for throughout the life cycle. In addition, at each stage of the material's life, there may also be qualitative environmental or health impacts that should be considered, such as the carbon emissions into the atmosphere, chemical leaching into water systems, VOC emissions in indoor environments, or environmental impacts at end of life with either recycling processes or landfill conditions. LCA tools are becoming more readily available for use during the building design process and can be used independently or integrated directly into Building Information Modeling (BIM) or other similar software platforms. Tally is one LCA tool that was developed by the architecture firm Kieran Timberlake and is able to be integrated with Autodesk software (K.T. Innovations, 2017). The challenge with most LCA tools is that the ability to produce accurate material accounting information is dependent on the databases that are available for the materials being studied for design integration. For examples, some material LCA databases are limited to typical construction materials such as concrete, steel, and wood framing members. Many LCA databases are not yet developed with regional specificity nor do most databases have other details that could impact the life cycle accounting (i.e., composite chemistries, finishes, sourcing variations, etc.). While the promise of integrating LCA into the building design process provides hope that we will be able to achieve better informed decision-making based on material impacts, especially with regard to the environmental and health effects, there is still a large amount of research required to bring these databases into relevancy for many specific construction contexts and for future and emerging building materials and methods.

Fisheye Lens Photos

The use of fisheye lens photography is a technique that emerged from the field of plant sciences with the study of tree canopies and their relative spread in relation to tree growth mechanisms (Macfarlane et al., 2007). The fisheye lens allows for the image capture of a 180-degree field of view, which fits into a full circle as a two-dimensional photograph. When two views are composited together from the same fixed camera location (i.e., view up and view down, or view forward and view backward), the result is a 360-degree field-of-view basis for the physical environment influencing the stationary point of the camera's position. The use of the fisheye lens photographs for architectural research was adapted for calculating view factors of the different materials and radiant conditions surrounding the position of a human in space. This is a method that is used to establish information needed in the MRT calculation that helps inform human thermal comfort. In addition, the fisheye lens photographs are also used to establish view factors of different VIS light conditions surrounding the position of a human to help inform glare analyses. Many architectural software platforms allow for fisheye lens images to be generated with the embedded rendering tools, allowing designers to analyze the thermal comfort and glare variables of materials and spaces in the design process.

Machine Learning Technologies

The concept of machine learning is one that requires computational techniques with embedded algorithms and the ongoing collection of data or information. Data and information are typically collected in real time via sensors, sensing devices, or human interface inputs. The data is then processed through a computation platform, which can be embedded in a microcontroller, for instance, or otherwise centrally located in an information technology system cloud or building management system (BMS) hub. Based on the learning algorithm defined for the data analysis, the output of the processing will describe an action, message, behavior, or change in a system function. Over time, the computational platform can be anticipatory and predictive in its messaging to the system based on the data it is receiving and its memory of similar patterns of historical data. Conceptually, the system is learning and adapting to specific conditions based on information and processing algorithms. Machine learning technologies, such as sensors and microcontrollers, are becoming more prevalent in both architectural design research and building implementation practices. The notion of smart buildings and smart cities is dependent on the decentralized deployment of sensors and data collection devices that can feed into computational platforms and build information databases. Many commercial technologies exist for smart building deployment including environmental control systems (lighting and thermal), security systems, water and air quality monitoring systems, as well as active façade components such as daylight control devices or smart glazing systems. However, these commercial technologies are proprietary and costly for architectural research, especially within small firms or educational contexts. Other more accessible and affordable devices, which can also be customized and adapted to unique conditions, are typically found through Arduino, Raspberry Pi, Particle, and Adafruit. These are vendors who specialize in microcontrollers, sensors, and related devices that can be integrated with data collection and computation platforms to provide machine learning or Internet of Things (IoT) functionality. At the Adaptive Environments Design Lab (AEDL) at the University of Arizona, an environmental test chamber is used to integrate different material system prototype studies with machine learning techniques. The sensing devices are incorporated on both sides of the chamber: one is for environmental input and represents outdoor design conditions, and the second chamber represents the controlled indoor environment. The sensors on both sides feed into a microcontroller and computation platform, which analyzes the data and feeds back a signal to an actuator for the material system prototype to engage in a change – for example, a pump might send water to the system to cause swelling of the modules and a concurrent change in heat capacitance and daylight transmission, or an electric charge might signal the polymer film to become more transparent or opaque for light and heat control. In the research process of adaptive material systems for human health and wellbeing, the integration of machine learning for system functions in corroboration with human experience biometrics is a goal for intelligent system design. This requires the material prototypes to be scaled up for human interaction testing, which takes place at the SensorLab at the University of Arizona, where human subjects can experience the environmental functions of the material systems and a conversation between biometric data and material prototype actuation can begin to take place (i.e., provide more or less humidity, light, or heat).

References

Aeroqual. (2019). Outdoor air monitoring equipment. Retrieved from https://www.aeroqual.com/outdoor-air-quality/outdoor-products

Ansaldo, M. (2019, July 24). The best indoor air-quality monitors: Identify the pollutants that can compromise your health and comfort. Retrieved from https://www.techhive.com/article/3356448/best-indoor-air-quality-monitor.html

Bandodkar, A. J., & Wang, J. (2014, July). Non-invasive wearable electrochemical sensors: A review. *Trends in Biotechnology, 32*(7), 363–371.

Banica, F. G. (2012). *Chemical Sensors and Biosensors: Fundamentals and Applications.* John Wiley & Sons, Chichester. http://dx.doi.org/10.1002/9781118354162

Capogrosso, M., Milekovic, T., Borton, D., Wagner, F., Moraud, E. M., Mignardot, J. B., ... & Rey, E. (2016). A brain–spine interface alleviating gait deficits after spinal cord injury in primates. *Nature, 539*(7628), 284–288.

Challoner, A., Pilla, F., & Gill, L. (2015, December). Prediction of indoor air exposure from outdoor air quality using an artificial neural network model for inner city commercial buildings. *International Journal of Environmental Research and Public Health, 12*(12), 15233–15253.

Clark, Leland C., & Lyons, Champ. (1962). Electrode systems for continuous monitoring in cardiovascular surgery. *Annals of the New York Academy of Sciences, 102*(1), 29–45.

Giri, T. K., Chakrabarty, S., & Ghosh, B. (2017, January 28). Transdermal reverse iontophoresis: A novel technique for therapeutic drug monitoring. *Journal of Controlled Release, 246,* 30–38.

Google. (n.d.). Google nest protect 2nd generation. Retrieved from https://store.google.com/us/product/nest_protect_2nd_gen

Hagedorn, J. G., Dunkers, J. P., Satterfield, S. G., Peskin, A. P., Kelso, J. T., & Terrill, J. E. (2007). Measurement tools for the immersive visualization environment: Steps toward the virtual laboratory. *Journal of research of the National Institute of Standards and Technology, 112*(5), 257.

International Well Building Institute (IWBI). (2017). 53. Visual lighting design. Retrieved from https://standard.wellcertified.com/v2/light/visual-lighting-design

Konis, K., Mack, W. J., & Schnieder, E. L. (2018, May 30). Pilot study to examine the effects of indoor daylight exposure on depression and other neuropsychiatric symptoms in people living with dementia in long-term care communities. *Clinical Interventions in Aging, 13,* 1071–1077.

K.T. Innovations. (2017). Tally version (2017). Retrieved from https://kierantimberlake.com/page/tally

Licea, M. (2018, May 19). North Americans lead other countries in time spent indoors. Retrieved from https://nypost.com/2018/05/19/north-americans-lead-other-countries-in-time-spent-indoors/

Lim, Ji Won, Ha, Dogyeong, Lee, Jongwan, Lee, Sung Kuk, & Kim, Taesung. (2015). Review of micro/nanotechnologies for microbial biosensors. *Frontiers in Bioengineering and Biotechnology,* 3, 61–61.

Lloyd, M. (2013). *Thermal imaging systems.* Springer Science & Business Media, Springer New York, NY.

Macfarlane, C., Grigg, A., & Evangelista, C. (2007). Estimating forest leaf area using cover and fullframe fisheye photography: Thinking inside the circle. *Agricultural and Forest Meteorology, 146*(1–2), 1–12.

Mulchandani, A., Rogers, K. R., & SpringerLink. (1998). *Enzyme and microbial biosensors techniques and protocols.* Humana Press, Humana Totowa, NJ.

Nikolić, D., Maftei, L., & Whyte, J. (2019). Becoming familiar: How infrastructure engineers begin to use collaborative virtual reality in their interdisciplinary practice. *Journal of Information Technology in Construction (ITcon), 24*(26), 489–508.

Norwood, M. F., Lakhani, A., Maujean, A., Zeeman, H., Creux, O. & Kendall, E. 2019. Brain activity, underlying mood and the environment: A systematic review. *Journal of Environmental Psychology, 65,* 101321.

Rizzo, A. (2003). A SWOT analysis of the field of virtual rehabilitation. In *Proceedings of the Second International Workshop on Virtual Rehabilitation* (pp. 1–2).

Runyon, J. R., Jia, M., Goldstein, M. R., Skeath, P., Abrell, L., Chorover, J., & Sternberg, E. M. (2019). Dynamic behavior of cortisol and cortisol metabolites in human eccrine sweat. *International Journal of Prognostics and Health Management, 10,* 1–11.

Sahin, L., & Figueiro, M. (2013). Alerting effects of short-wavelength (blue) and long-wavelength (red) lights in the afternoon. *Physiology & Behavior, 116–117,* 1–7.

Sensirion: The Sensor Company. (2020). Environmental sensors. Retrieved from https://www.sensirion.com/en/environmental-sensors/

Stieve, Hennig. (1983). Sensors of biological organisms — biological transducers. *Sensors and Actuators, 4,* 689–704.

Tierney, M. J., Tamada, J. A., Potts, R. O., et al. (2001, December). Clinical evaluation of GlucoWatch biographer: A continual, non-invasive glucose monitor for patients with diabetes. *Biosensors and Bioelectronics, 16*(9–12), 621–629.

UC San Diego. (2013, April 18). Biosensor tattoo monitors sweat for health indicators. Retrieved from https://jacobsschool.ucsd.edu/news/news_releases/release.sfe?id=1353

Ullrich, S. (2005). Mechanisms underlying UV-induced immune suppression. *Mutation Research/Fundamental and Molecular Mechanisms of Mutagenesis, 571*(1–2), 185–205.

UV Radiation. (2019, May 20). Retrieved from https://www.cdc.gov/features/uv-radiation-safety/index.html

Velux. (n.d.). Daylight calculations and measurements. Retrieved from https://www.velux.com/deic/daylight/daylight-calculations-and-measurements

Wessels, P. W., & Basten, T. G. H. (2016, September). Design aspects of acoustic noise sensor networks for environmental noise monitoring. *Applied Acoustics, 110,* 227–234.

Yin, M., Borton, D. A., Komar, J., Agha, N., Lu, Y., Li, H., ... & Larson, L. (2014). Wireless neurosensor for full-spectrum electrophysiology recordings during free behavior. *Neuron, 84*(6), 1170–1182.

Zadeh, R. S., Shepley, M. M., & Williams, G. (2014, July 1). The impact of windows and daylight on acute-care nurses' physiological, psychological, and behavioral health. *HERD: Health Environments Research & Design Journal, 7*(4), 35–61.

6 Design and Analysis Methods

Introduction

The design and analysis methods that we engage as architects and researchers of the built environment inform the type of results that will emerge. Our discussion in this chapter is organized around two themes: design platforms and measurement methods. In the first section, we discuss how existing design platforms such as Building Information Modeling (BIM) and parametric three-dimensional (3D) software can be accessed and enhanced to inform human health and wellbeing outcomes in the design process. We also present virtual reality (VR) environments and Internet of Things (IoT) – two emerging areas of study, including their integration platforms.

Design Platforms

VR Environments

The role of VR in architecture has become increasingly important in the design process and has the potential to become integral in transforming the industry (Figure 6.1). The ability of VR to transform a building design into a fully interactive 3D environment gives the audience an accurate physical representation of a building's floor plan. A major challenge for building design is translating the idea of a model to a fully developed building; VR can be beneficial in this respect since it brings clients in collaboration with the design process. For example, a complete and detailed representation of a building design that clients can see will make the process of feedback more straightforward. Being able to fully interact constitutes being able to open and close doors and move objects throughout the room. In addition, the ability to picture real-world scenarios in a virtual world will also be more easily translated into the real world to anticipate errors or missing considerations in advance to create safer and user-friendly environments (TMD Studio LTD, 2020) (Figure 6.1).

VR software is also very accessible because it can be downloaded onto most smartphone devices (TMD Studio LTD, 2020). The ability of VR to

DOI: 10.4324/9780367814748-9

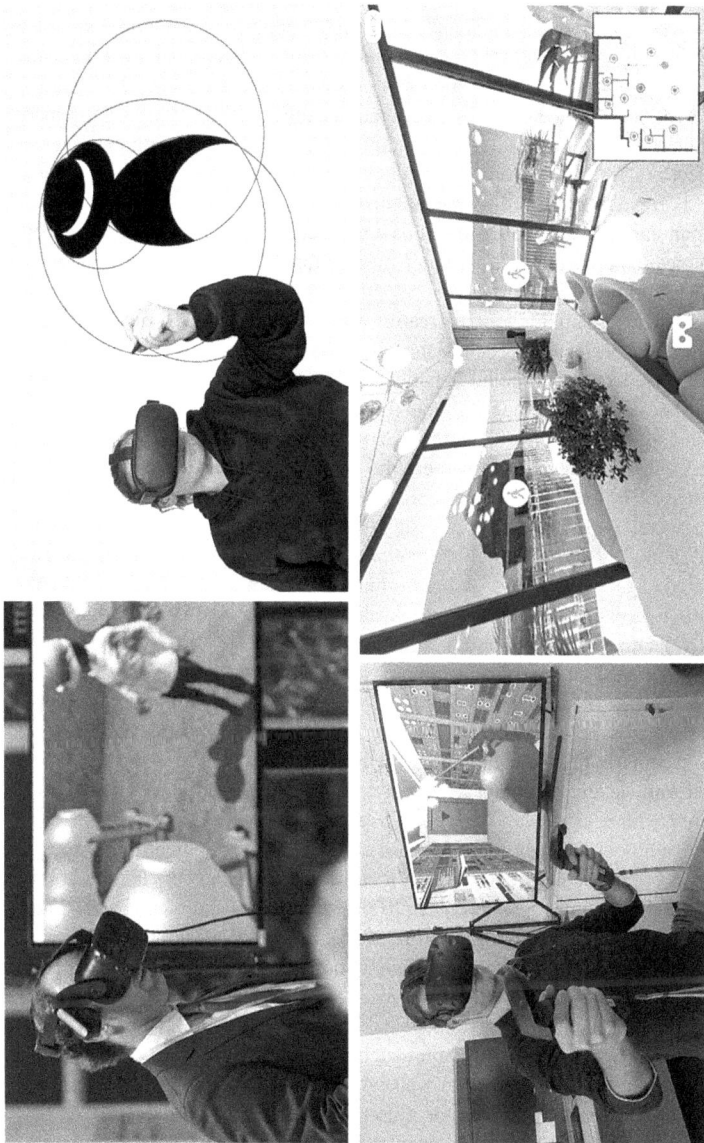

Figure 6.1 Composite Images: Virtual reality Environments.

create immersive environments for participants increases the potential to measure and anticipate health and wellbeing outcomes. This can be done by making detailed behavioral observations and taking physiological measurements by noninvasive wearable devices simultaneously in real time. Examples of these physiological measurements include stress and relaxation responses, activity, and sleep quality which can be tracked continuously. This data directly informs solutions for better human health, wellness, and performance, and is therefore very valuable. By implementing VR into design practices to reflect real-world environments, both therapeutic and healing environments can be readily produced. Little is known, however, about how VR can aid design and medical professionals as a preoccupancy evaluation tool for best practices and whether it is a reliable method for reflecting human responses to a real-world environment.

VR can potentially help in creating a therapeutic environment for populations with special needs such as the elderly and disabled. VR has been used to reduce anxiety and agitation in patients with Alzheimer's disease. This is possible because of its unique ability to fully immerse the patient in a specific controlled environment. Uwajeh et al. (2019) utilized a VR headset with its visual and auditory features to show peaceful beach scenes, forests, and animals to patients. The results revealed a significant improvement in patients' moods and overall experiences. Studies such as these indicate that the VR technique may allow for more detailed behavioral observations which can be directly related to stress, wellness, and performance. The ability of VR to provide patients with a sense of therapeutic peace is unique and also indicative of its potential that can lead to higher return on investment (ROI) for organizations.

VR is still an emerging technology in medicine, but it is becoming increasingly accessible and affordable. Overcoming physical limitations is imperative to a person with a disability. Another advantage of VR, therefore, could be its ability to help people with disabilities by enabling them to expand their knowledge and skills while staying in place. Smartphone applications paired with a cardboard headset are readily accessible and affordable, and these are now the only two pieces of software and equipment that a person needs to explore a virtual world. VR, in this manner, has the unique ability to help disabled people overcome physical limitations and break barriers that were previously beyond reach (NPR, 2015). Learning new things with limited movement would have been previously inaccessible without the use of VR. By being able to navigate a virtual world without the same limitations they experience in their immediate physical environment, people with disabilities can learn a variety of new hobbies such as learning how to surf even though they do not have the ability to walk. Additionally, VR can be personalized, safe, and relatively risk-free for a user (Corporate Learning Trends, 2018). The ability of VR to be customized and bridge different groups and populations with special needs makes it an important emerging technology that can be used therapeutically, medically, architecturally.

BIM Platforms

BIM platforms are digital tools that allow for the integration of data with 3D architectural and engineering drawings. BIM models are descriptive with quantitative information about the contents embedded in the design. The metrics might describe the counts of material or product quantities that are informative when developing cost estimates for construction, or the metrics might describe the environmental impact of certain materials (such as in the life cycle assessment (LCA)) included in the proposed design. While BIM models originated primarily for use by the Architecture, Engineering, and Construction (AEC) industry to provide construction cost information about the project through its 3D components in the design model (Kensek, 2014), the conceptual framework of BIM has evolved to encompass other information modeling benefits.

BIM platforms also allow for the interoperability of data-rich 3D digital models with various databases and other tools. Many BIM tools are very specific to environmental performance analyses, such as daylighting analysis, airflow analysis, or building energy analysis. Some examples of BIM platforms for environmental information include Autodesk's Green Building Studio, IES's Green Solutions, Bentley's Hevacomp, and various tools offered open source by the Department of Energy (DOE) such as EnergyPlus and eQuest (Lu et al., 2017). The evolving field of BIM tools and its array of platforms is sometimes challenged through application programming interface (API) links, which need to be created by software developers to ensure the interoperability of the different BIM models and analysis platforms.

One area for BIM that is not yet explored or developed is an integrated analysis for health and wellbeing, which is a promising area for consideration in future software platforms. Though we are able to obtain data on human visual and thermal comfort metrics through our digital design models, we are yet to more fully understand the health and wellbeing implications of a given spatial configuration in conjunction with its occupancy patterns and the correlated environmental and material aspects. As we see performance metrics characterized and established through entities such as the WELL standard, we will also begin to see the opportunity to translate these types of information inputs and outputs in our 3D modeling environments.

Parametric 3D Design

Parametric modeling is a method by which the design of spatial and material conditions can result from testing different informational inputs to the model. Parametric 3D design is now a common method of digital modeling, where various inputs such as environmental information or volumetric conditions are utilized as the constraints and/or adjustable measures that will inform resulting object morphology, surface configuration, or spatial conditions, for example.

It requires a different set of procedures in the digital design process in comparison with traditional computer-aided design (CAD) drawing, which are driven by vector-based outputs of lines, arcs, and polylines. User to work behind the scenes, of the digital content by developing code-based logical arguments in the platform's syntax to produce operational constraints and modulation controls. For example, a sphere could be drawn in CAD with a "sphere tool" or parametrically by defining the 3D coordinates of the sphere, such as its center point and diameter, radius, or volume. In the CAD model, any adjustments to the design of the sphere need to be manually conducted with editing tools, such as scaling or moving or cropping. However, in the parametric model, the design of the sphere can now be driven by its information inputs – if the desire is to obtain a certain volume, the volume can be defined with a number slider input, or the volume might be further defined by the analysis of some other variables such as heat gain or daylight access. Parametric 3D design allows for a much more intelligent flow and process of integrating evidence-based information and simulation analyses for the aspects of the environment that will more often impact our human health and wellbeing. Furthermore, the parameters of any parametric design are fully defined through the agency of the model's author(s) and a decision-based logic, so the results incorporate designer agency as well as intelligence.

One can imagine the power of parametric 3D modeling with health and wellbeing measures in the design process. The basis of a spatial configuration, its material compositions, and environmental performance could be determined through human health inputs such as biometric variable that require specific light levels, temperatures, and occupancy patterns to allow for optimized wellbeing across temporal instances. The parametric platform that is widely used in the architecture design field is through Grasshopper, the coding logic platform, which is linked with Rhino, the 3D modeling environment. Grasshopper incorporates numerous plug-ins that allow for different facets of parametric design, such as physics-based modeling engines or interfaces with energy modeling engines. The possibility for customization is seemingly endless and accessible for those only semi-familiar with coding languages. Because of the power of Grasshopper as a robust platform for numerous parametric tools, other industry software applications now incorporate similar parametric options such as the beta version Parametric Modeler for Sketchup or Autodesk's Inventor software. Unlike typical 3D software platforms that are object driven, the parametric platforms are driven by information, similar to reverse engineering in a BIM model.

IoT Integration Platforms

The ever-expanding world of data collection through distributed sensors and devices is feeding into an engine that is described as the IoT. IoT is a relatively broad term referring to the combination of technologies, embedded systems, networking, and information technology (Iqbal, 2020). IoT is a combination of the accumulative electronic objects that function in different ways while being connected with a network so that the functions of the objects might be informed by specific data or otherwise are collecting and feeding data back to a centralized server or cloud-based engine. Smartphones are the most accessible examples of an IoT device – our cell phones must be connected to a network, whether through Wi-Fi or cellular connections, to perform certain activities like displaying new email, text messages, or webpages. In addition, our smartphones can feed data back to a network if we allow such features to be enabled. For example, if our smartphone is tracking the number of steps we make each day, that data can be stored on a cloud server and retrieved at a future time. That same data about our steps per day might also serve to initiate messages or notices back to us about our health, such as reminders to take a few more steps before the day ends or a note of achievement. When we consider the array of biometric devices that are discussed in the previous chapters and the ability for vast amounts of real-time human health sensing data acquisition, in combination with environmental sensing data collection within and around building spaces, the field of IoT is certainly becoming highly applicable for playing a significant role in the future of our wellbeing in the built environment. To revisit the building management system (BMS) for instance (the centralized brain for environmental controls in a building), the potential for the BMS to integrate occupant biometric data and provide real-time responsive actuation of environmental system adjustments to accommodate improved wellbeing is possible. Currently, we find that BMS for energy and water conservation processes in buildings is integrated to the management portfolios of Operation and Maintenance (O&M) costs. However, the BMS might incorporate anonymous biometrics from its occupants to establish the wellbeing processes in buildings that can inform comparable portfolios for both O&M costs and ROI data. IoT can be integrated on a smaller scale as well. Rather than expanded to a building or entire city, localized embedded biosensors and environmental controls can allow for human-scale responsive systems to function and operate, which occurs through machine-learning processes (described in Chapter 2.2).

Measurement Methods

Correlational Data Analysis

Correlational methods are useful for analyzing the potential cause-and-effect relationships across variant phenomena. Correlational data analysis often requires the use of graphs, charts, maps, or other visualization tools to assess the relationships between datasets. Correlational analysis is traditionally considered a quantitative research method, but qualitative data can also be utilized for correlational studies. Correlational data analysis methods are utilized frequently in the field of psychology, thus providing an informative tool for studying the influence of built environment on human wellbeing and psychological effects.

The fundamentals of correlational data analysis are based on rules and terminology of statistics. Some of the correlational data analysis methods include Bayesian, Pearson's, meta-analysis, sequential, observational, and polychoric. The data being analyzed might come in different forms, such as ordinal data or a neural network. Other terms characterize certain conditions of a dataset, such as an effect size benchmark which indicates the meaningfulness of the relationship between data variables.

ROI Analysis

Translating human health research findings into built environment outcomes is important from an ROI perspective. The various design platforms discussed in this chapter can be used to analyze ROI, which is key information for stakeholders in government agencies and private industry. Case studies that research the impact of building designs on human health in this regard can benefit ROI since they reveal the potential of research outcomes to improve worker productivity and performance. From the LCA perspective, personnel salaries take a significant portion of the cost of a building and even a small amount of productivity and performance improvement will easily justify, for example, a renovation. For example, a study by Ghahramani et al. (2019) analyzed the impact of carbon dioxide (CO_2) on work performance and overall health outcomes. This study was performed in an office work environment, and the employees wore wearable air quality sensors on their face and chest. The study concluded that there is a CO_2 bubble that lingers if one sits in one place for a long period of time. Previous studies have revealed that high CO_2 concentrations may negatively impact cognition, performance, and overall employee health (Allen et al., 2015). The researchers of this study deduced that an installation of desk fans near the workers would help deplete the CO_2 bubbles that build up near the office workers (Ghahramani et al., 2019). In addition to desk fans, from an architecture perspective, better designs for work stations and spatial layouts could also combat this phenomenon. An ROI analysis could then be performed by measuring the change in employee productivity and performance and comparing it to the cost of such a research study and subsequent design and construction costs. In addition, studies have shown that the amount of sick leave an employee takes can be reduced by proper ventilation in a school or work environment. When there are lower levels of indoor air pollutants, workers are more inclined to take shorter amounts of sick leave, and they also have the potential to be more productive (Milton et al., 2000). Similarly, Clements-Croome et al. (2008) looked at the effects of ventilation in classroom environments. Increased CO_2 levels and poor indoor air quality were found to have a negative effect on student performance. High levels of CO_2 could cause students to be less attentive. To counter this, they found that a small portable ventilator supplying fresh outside air and placed in each classroom was effective. Quantifying amounts of sick leave and absenteeism in office workers, or student attentiveness and performance both before and after research and design interventions, therefore, could be another accurate method of performing an ROI analysis.

Using noninvasive wearable devices to measure physiological health could also assist with ROI studies. From an employer's perspective, an additional incentive to provide healthy and comfortable work environments is that healthy employees ultimately perform better and have a higher chance of remaining loyal to the company they are working for (Muaremi et al., 2013). Muaremi et al. (2013) analyzed the information acquired from smartphones and wearable chest belts in workers to assess stress throughout the work day. Specifically, during the work day, they collected audio, physical activity, and communication data. Furthermore, they collected heart rate variability (HRV) data at night. Collecting data on stress and giving employees an opportunity to acknowledge their stress while giving them the tools to recover is known to be imperative for leading a healthy work environment life. The researchers, therefore, developed a smartphone application that monitored employee stress. They found that excessive workload was one of the major reasons for inducing stress in employees which could ultimately lead to them quitting their jobs (Muaremi et al., 2013). This study is another example of how monitoring the stress in a workplace environment can be a good model for demonstrating the impact on ROI for employers.

These studies reveal how identifying and creating a healthy built environment framework through research and design interventions can lead an overall gain on money invested, that is, ROI. Effective ROI analysis information can help businesses and organizations make a case for investing in healthy environments to work and live in, which ultimately gives them incentive to make a real-world impact on the built environment.

Stress, Wellbeing, and Performance

There is a clear link between individuals' physical health and the levels of stress they experience. Acute and chronic stressors – both environment and nonenvironment related – can have negative impacts on human health. Bioresponsive material systems and wearable technologies that are continuously linked to the internet can help a researcher analyze stress that is directly related to human wellbeing and performance. There has been an emergence of wearable technologies – examples of which have been discussed in this book – that can use heart rate activity and skin conductance to monitor and identify stress levels in individuals. Using wearable technologies to aid in detecting stress during daily activities may help discover the causes of major stressors in the built environment and subsequently reduce or eliminate them for better health and wellbeing outcomes (Can et al., 2019).

A common subjective method to measure stress is by using questionnaires that ask people to quantify their mood. Muaremi et al. (2013) assessed a more effective way to measure stress by combining subjective methods with objective means by using a smartphone application and a wearable heart monitor to evaluate HRV. HRV is a measurement of the autonomic nervous system and can be effectively analyzed to indicate stress, leading to potential associations between health disorders and stress. This study highlights how using smartphone applications and measuring overall HRV by using a wearable device can be effective in identifying stress and relating it to environmental factors – a method which is more reliable and less subjective than a typical questionnaire (Muaremi et al., 2013). Moreover, detecting stress at early stages is important for future individual health and wellbeing.

A number of advanced technologies are being produced to help older adults in both physical and mental aspects of their daily lives. Vulnerable populations such as older adults, however, experience significant limitations in the way that they may use VR or wearable technologies to help facilitate an improved quality of life. Older adults may be reluctant to utilize these technologies because of the fear of stigmatization. VR or other wearable devices that bear a resemblance to a health assistance device could be indicative of a frail, weak, or ill older adult which may translate into an unwillingness to use them (Lee et al., 2019). Further, elderly individuals may consider a wearable device invasive or troublesome. However, ambient intelligence aims to take the negative connotation of wearable devices on the elderly and make their home an environment that can monitor and enhance their health and wellbeing. It makes their environments customizable and responsive, with the ability to monitor health and provide social communication, companionship or recreation, and entertainment (Grossi et al., 2019). The development of smart homes for older adults by using this technology is significant from a health and built environment perspective.

References

Allen, J. G., MacNaughton, P., Satish, U., Santanam, S., Vallarino, J., & Spengler, J. D. (2015). Associations of cognitive function scores with carbon dioxide, ventilation, and volatile organic compound exposures in office workers: A controlled exposure study of green and conventional office environments. *Environmental Health Perspectives, 124*(6), 805–812.

Can, Y. S., Chalabianloo, N., Ekiz, D., & Ersoy, C. (2019). Continuous stress detection using wearable sensors in real life: Algorithmic programming contest case study. *Sensors, 19*(8), 1849.

Clements-Croome, D., Awbi, H., Bako-Biro, Z., Kochhar, N., & Williams, M. (2008). Ventilation rates in schools. *Building and Environment, 43*(3), 362–367.

Corporate Learning Trends. (2018, May 17). GAAD: How virtual reality can transform the way people with disabilities learn. Retrieved from https://www.d2l.com/corporate/blog/gaad-virtual-reality-people-disabilities-learn/

Ghahramani, A., Pantelic, J., Vannucci, M., Pistore, L., Liu, S., Gilligan, B., ... & Sternberg, E. (2019). Personal CO_2 bubble: Context-dependent variations and wearable sensors usability. *Journal of Building Engineering, 22*, 295–304.

Grossi, G., Lanzarotti, R., Napoletano, P., Noceti, N., & Odone, F. (2019). Positive technology for elderly wellbeing: A review. *Pattern Recognition Letters*, Volume 137, p. 61–70.

Iqbal, Hussain, Huanlai, Imran, Hussain, Sajjad, Huanlai, Xing, & Imran, Muhammad A. (2020). *Enabling the internet of things: Fundamentals, design, and applications* (1st ed.). John Wiley & Sons, Ltd: Hoboken, NJ.

Kensek, K. M. (2014). *Building information modeling*. ProQuest Ebook Central, London.

Lee, L. N., Kim, M. J., & Hwang, W. J. (2019). Potential of augmented reality and virtual reality technologies to promote wellbeing in older adults. *Applied Sciences, 9*(17), 3556.

Lu, Y., Wu, Z., Chang, R., & Li, Y. (2017). Building information modeling (BIM) for green buildings: A critical review and future directions. *Automation in Construction, 83*, 134–148.

Milton, D. K., Glencross, P. M., & Walters, M. D. (2000). Abstract. *Indoor Air, 10*(4), 212–221.

Muaremi, A., Arnrich, B., & Tröster, G. (2013). Towards measuring stress with smartphones and wearable devices during workday and sleep. *BioNanoScience, 3*(2), 172–183.

NPR (National Public Radio). (2015, October 22). Affordable virtual reality opens new worlds for people with disabilities. Retrieved from https://www.npr.org/sections/health-shots/2015/10/22/450573400/affordable-virtual-reality-opens-new-worlds-for-people-with-disabilities

TMD Studio LTD. (2020, February 1). Virtual reality uses in architecture and design. Retrieved from https://medium.com/studiotmd/virtual-reality-uses-in-architecture-and-design-c5d54b7c1e89

Uwajeh, Patrick Chukwuemeke et al. "Therapeutic gardens as a design approach for optimising the healing environment of patients with Alzheimer's disease and other dementias: A narrative review." *Explore* (New York, N.Y.) vol. 15,5 (2019): 352–362. doi:10.1016/j.explore.2019.05.002

Part III
Applications
Case Studies and Future Directions

7   Case Studies

Introduction

This chapter discusses a set of case study projects from research and design practices that demonstrate the tools, techniques, and methods introduced in this book. These case studies are discussed in detail with an explanation of their representation across the range of built environment impacts on human health and wellbeing.

Case Studies

Studies conducted by researchers in universities, government agencies, and the building and health industry, pertaining to the built environment and its impact on human wellbeing, are evaluated and discussed as case studies in this chapter. These organizations and their studies were chosen because of their use of state-of-the-art emerging and advanced technologies in the field, which drive the research on human health and wellbeing outcomes. The issues discussed by these case studies range from emerging technologies' health facilities to health equity and social issues in health design (Figure 7.1). These concerns are significant since they inform the design and construction of built environments which directly impact human health, productivity, and performance.

The Center for Health Facilities Design and Testing

The Center for Health Facilities Design and Testing at Clemson University primarily focuses on improving technological aspects of design and health research and integrating them into built environments to improve health outcomes. Goals include building a network of researchers to address safety issues by analyzing the physical environment, supporting design innovation, and integrating research, practice, and education through real-world projects. They use a variety of tools and technologies to accomplish this goal. Some of their current projects involve using virtual reality (VR) and a variety of

DOI: 10.4324/9780367814748-11

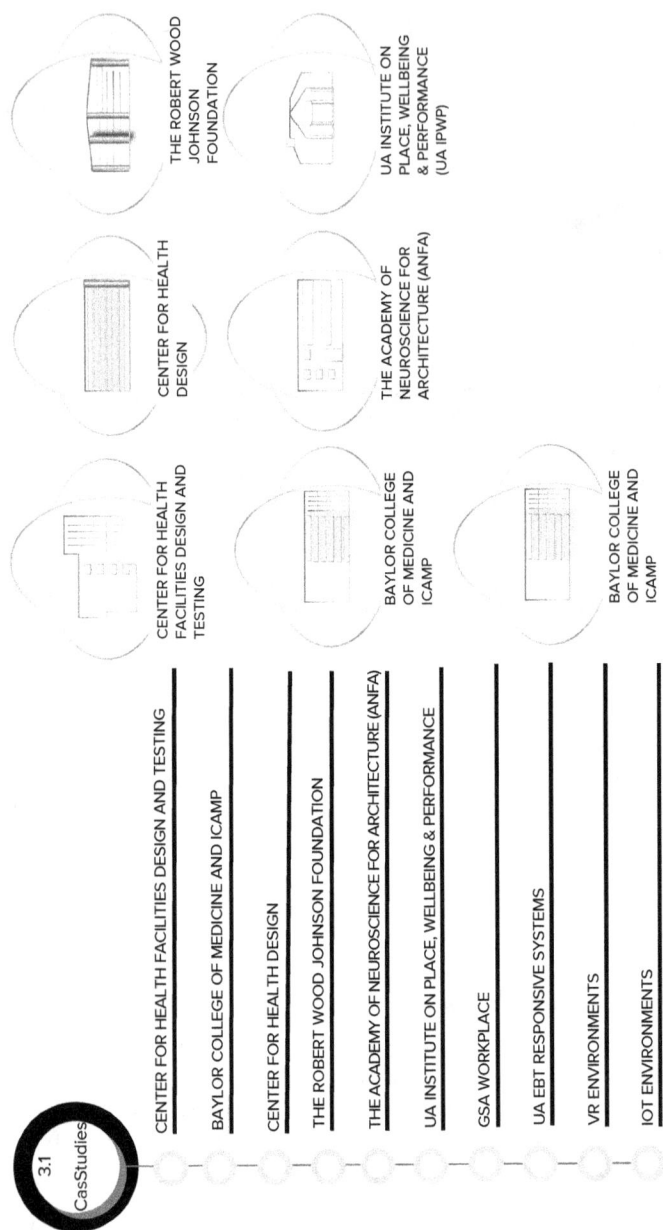

CENTER FOR HEALTH FACILITIES DESIGN AND TESTING

BAYLOR COLLEGE OF MEDICINE AND ICAMP

CENTER FOR HEALTH DESIGN

THE ROBERT WOOD JOHNSON FOUNDATION

THE ACADEMY OF NEUROSCIENCE FOR ARCHITECTURE (ANFA)

UA INSTITUTE ON PLACE, WELLBEING & PERFORMANCE

GSA WORKPLACE

UA EBT RESPONSIVE SYSTEMS

VR ENVIRONMENTS

IOT ENVIRONMENTS

Figure 7.1 Composite Diagram: Comparative Workplace Environment Examples of Research Settings.

tool kits such as the safe operating room (OR), the Clemson health-care work system ergonomic assessment, and the ambulatory care center design which focuses on improving patient care, designing waiting rooms and surgical environments, and preventing falls with technology-based interventions. These advanced tools and technologies aid in the important research they do surrounding design innovation (Clemson University, 2019).

One of the Center's significant current projects is titled *Designing Waiting Rooms in Surgical Environments, the Impact of the Layout of the Waiting Area and the Design of Seating*. The goal of this project is to improve an individual's waiting experience. The study focuses on the impact of furniture location on various tasks ranging from patient check-in, to receiving a phone call, getting coffee, and waiting for surgery to end. This study holds much significance in the field of health-care design because it investigates the significance of the built environment on human comfort while utilizing VR to examine the different environmental attributes that impact common tasks in a waiting area (Clemson University, 2019). The benefits of VR are very apparent in this study design because it exemplifies the ability of VR to engage its audience in the visualization of different building designs, spatial layouts, and characteristics (Nikolić et al., 2019).

Baylor College of Medicine and Interdisciplinary Consortium on Advanced Motion Performance

Baylor College of Medicine and the Interdisciplinary Consortium on Advanced Motion Performance (iCAMP) lab focus on technological advancements in design for health and wellbeing, specifically innovations in sensing, mobility, and VR. The main goal of this lab is to conduct impactful research in surgical disease to improve treatment and quality of life for patients by improving stability, healing, and mobility. This lab uses a variety of innovative sensing and measuring technology such as body-worn sensors (also commonly referred to as wearable technologies) along with ancillary technologies such as VR, thermal imaging, and artificial intelligence. In addition, they utilize smart signal processing to identify physical activity patterns, spatiotemporal parameters of gait, balance, and three-dimensional joint kinematics and kinetics. They aim to develop several novel metrics which are fundamental to define disease state, assess motor learning and motor-cognitive decline, and determine biomechanical variabilities by extracting the most relevant information from human motion. They conduct research that is local to their lab as well as partner with a variety of businesses, analysts, and international research teams to advance the field of motion performance (Baylor College of Medicine, 2020).

The current projects by the Baylor College of Medicine involve research using different emerging technologies which include wearable devices and environmental sensors, and the use of VR, wearable technologies, thermal imaging, and artificial intelligence to help improve mobility, stability, and healing worldwide. For example, in one project, the iCAMP team is using wearable sensors to measure walking and to assess the severity of neurogenic disorders in supervised and free-living conditions (Baylor College of Medicine, 2020). This use of VR in projects such as these also reveals the value of this technology to measure health and wellbeing outcomes and highlights how this technology is being expanded by researchers worldwide. By collecting information that can be analyzed and in the generation of user-friendly design solutions at the predesign and preoccupancy phase, VR holds much potential in current and future health-related design research.

Center for Health Design

The Center for Health Design is a nonprofit research organization that focuses on evidence-based health-care facility design. It aims to create health-care facilities that promote healthier environments for both their patients and their staff. By empowering health-care leaders, researchers are able to conduct relevant research to improve health outcomes, optimize the patient experience of care, and increase health-care provider and staff satisfaction and performance through quality design. By stressing the benefits of investing in health facility through research, the Center for Health Design plays a key role in encouraging the advancement and practice in health-care design. Researchers in the Center use a variety of tools and technologies to conduct their projects and realize their outcomes. They offer a variety of services which include identification, custom development, validation, virtual training, on-site training of tools, analysis of electronic health record systems, robotic surgeries, remote video connections, and medication safety systems (The Center for Health Design, 2020).

The Research Coalition at the Center for Health Design comprises research professionals, design practitioners, health-care administrators, and a diverse range of professionals from other related fields that can help guide their projects. State-of-the-art technologies are used and integrated into their research design to achieve their goal of creating improved health-care facilities and patient-centered care. The Research Coalition produces evidence-based research that will also ultimately contribute to safer and more effective health-care settings. Further, their architect members are committed to performing effective research on clinical outcomes and patient and staff satisfaction to create optimal healing environments (The Center for Health Design, 2020).

The Robert Wood Johnson Foundation

The Robert Wood Johnson Foundation (RWJF) funds a grant program that aims to discover, explore, and spread model interventions in health and wellbeing, and conduct meaningful research and evaluation. This philanthropic organization focuses on health systems, healthy communities, healthy children and families, and leadership for better health. It funds a wide variety of research to help address these concerns with an emphasis on aspects of health equity and social issues in health design. Its primary goal is to identify the major causes for health disparities in the United States by funding researchers whose work can build healthier and more equitable communities and providing evidence for actual policy change and practice (The Robert Wood Johnson Foundation, 2018).

RWJF aims to expand the nation's knowledge on the multitude of factors that have an impact on human health and influence health policy changes at a systemic level. Identifying the root causes of health inequality and disparities is crucial since this can inform potential solutions to improve the overall health and wellbeing of every individual. RWJF plays a significant role in this work (The Robert Wood Johnson Foundation, 2018).

The Academy of Neuroscience for Architecture

The primary mission of the Academy of Neuroscience for Architecture (ANFA) is to advance knowledge that links neuroscience research with human responses to built environments. The ANFA Hay Grant Research Program encourages researchers to analyze the connection between neuroscience and architecture and how the incorporation of neuroscience research can lead to healthy building designs. The John Paul Eberhard Fellowship, also given out by ANFA, solidifies its mission of promoting neuroscience to influence the design of the built environment by encouraging interdisciplinary graduate students (Masters and PhD) to create more linkages between architecture and neuroscience. One example of a relevant research topic suitable for a grant from ANFA would be analyzing the effects of artificial lighting on brain regulation and circadian rhythms. The primary goals of ANFA's programs are to research the impacts of architecture on neuroscience and provide evidence-based results to connect the two. ANFA also hosts an annual conference in which professionals, academics, and researchers in both fields and other related areas convene to present their latest work, share ideas, and discuss collaboration and future research possibilities (The Academy of Neuroscience for Architecture, 2020).

UA IPWP Workplace Human Performance and Health

The University of Arizona Institute on Place, Wellbeing & Performance (UA IPWP) links the University of Arizona College of Medicine, the Andrew Weil Center for Integrative Medicine (AWCIM), and the University of Arizona College of Architecture, Planning, and Landscape Architecture to focus on how human health is impacted by the built environment. The overarching mission of UA IPWP is to research and quantify stress, health, and wellbeing outcomes by working with practitioners, government agencies, corporations, and the community to create actual changes in policy that could make a difference and maximize productivity, creativity, and wellbeing (UA IPWP, 2019).

By university-wide, national, and international partnerships, UA IPWP provides design guidance for the objective of wellbeing. With 90% of time spent indoors, this research is valuable because little is known about how environmental conditions and designs impact human health and wellbeing (UA IPWP, 2019).

One example of UA IPWP's projects is its concept for the *Rooms for Wellbeing*, an interactive and immersive exhibit for the American Institute of Architects (AIA) Conference on Architecture in 2016. This exhibit gave visitors an opportunity to experience latest and emerging technologies for wearable devices and environmental sensors to measure the impact of the built environment on human health. Environmental attributes such as temperature, light, sound, and indoor air quality were measured to connect human behavioral, psychological, and behavioral responses. This exhibit demonstrated the significance of research on health and the built environment and its potential to help inform building standards that can help develop healthier physical environments (UA IPWP, 2019).

Another key project of UA IPWP is the Multimodal Objective Sensing to Assess Individuals with Context (MOSAIC) program run by the Intelligence Advanced Research Projects Activity (IARPA), a federal agency under the Director of National Intelligence. As part of MOSAIC, IPWP partnered with Lockheed Martin Advanced Technology Laboratories (LM ATL) to develop the Rapid Automatic & Adaptive Model of Performance Prediction (RAAMP2) system, a multimodal automated tool that reliably predicts human work performance with unobtrusive wearable and environmental sensors. RAAMP2 utilizes data provided by these sensors in a workplace environment, and 300 office workers measured continuously, in real time over a period of two months. This research program is in its phase and has so far revealed exciting possibilities to define individuals' health, wellbeing, and performance by linking real-time human physiological, behavioral, and psychological responses to real-time environmental measures. UA IPWP and LM ATL are currently working on manuscripts to publish these exciting findings in peer-reviewed journals (Office of the Director of National Intelligence, 2017; UA IPWP, 2019).

The US General Services Administration Workplace

The US General Services Administration (GSA) has successfully partnered with the UA IPWP, and Aclima Inc. – a company that manufactures wearable and environmental sensors – on research studies about performance and productivity in workplace environments. This partnership is a good example of a collaboration between government, industry, and academia to create healthy environments using state-of-the-art advanced technologies and sensing methods. Specifically, the goal of this study is to use environmental sensing technologies to map and measure temperature, sound, air quality, light, and other pertinent environmental attributes in real time to study the impact on human health and work performance. Advanced sensing technologies are used to analyze the influence of building design and spatial layout and characteristics on health and wellbeing. The sensors monitor different physiological aspects of workers such as heart activity, physical movement, and sleep activity. This objective data is combined with subjective data in the form of daily survey responses. By applying these advanced and emerging sensing technologies along with subjective perceptions and experiences of participants, researchers have data that can allow them to discover how different office conditions can affect the physical and mental health and wellbeing of office workers. Office workers are at an increased risk to illnesses because of sedentary behavior and design of their immediate work environments. The findings of this research, therefore, can positively influence the performance of office workers by reducing workplace absenteeism, illnesses, stress, and poor sleep quality directly associated with the work environment. The ultimate goal of such interdisciplinary teams is to make the workplace environments suitable for employees to thrive and not just survive (UA IPWP, 2019).

UA AEDL Responsive Systems and Sensing Lab

The University of Arizona (UA) Adaptive Environments Design Lab (AEDL) includes prototype development of bio-responsive material systems and emerging environmental building technologies. Once fabricated, the prototypes are then implemented for human interaction testing at the UA Sensing Lab in the College of Medicine. A couple of case example responsive system's prototypes with integrated sensing and human interaction testing include the BENCH and SHAPE projects. BENCH is a Biorhythmic Evaporative-cooling Nano-teCH membrane that is applied to a Computer Numerical Control (CNC) wood frame seating apparatus for human interaction testing. The interactive sensing function responds to the weight of a human body when seated on the bench, which actuates the peristaltic pumps to send water into the evaporative-cooling membrane. The idea is that the humidity in the immediate environment surrounding human occupants can provide a cooling effect and also calibrate the desired humidity levels for respiratory health. The BENCH is being set up in the UA's Sensing Lab, where ongoing human interaction testing with integrated biometric sensors can take place. The SHAPE prototype is a Soundscape with Hydrogel-Actuated Podium Electronics that incorporates wavelength specific sensors embedded in a hydrogel medium to assess proximities of human bodies to actuate sound and light performances. The SHAPE prototype will also be tested at the UA Sensing Lab and will allow for assessment of different sound and light performances on human stress response and relief, providing insight into how built environments and their material systems might incorporate multiple sensory functions for human wellbeing.

VR Environments

VR is defined as a three-dimensional technological medium that allows users to view a computer-generated environment through a head-mounted display (Jerdan et al., 2018). Previous chapters in this book have also described VR as both an area for healing through the immersive physical environment and a measurement tool that enables researchers to determine the overall impact of the built environment on human health and wellbeing. VR environments have been found to impact human health because they change the way humans interact with their immediate environment, essentially allowing individuals to perceive items within it and engage them. In this manner, VR leads to the design of interactive, safe, and healing environments. VR, therefore, as a design and research tool, is increasingly being used by researchers who focus on the relationship between human health and the built environment. Since VR is starting to become such an important method within the health-care field with the diverse ability to diagnose, rehabilitate, treat, and counsel patients, the work described in these case studies are imperative for future design implications for human health and wellbeing. An overarching goal of implementing emerging technologies such as VR can be their ability to help improve the design of environments inhabited by regular as well as special populations worldwide.

Internet of Things Environments

Sensors can act as if sensory systems in the human body in a building. Specifically, they are capable of recognizing a certain physical phenomenon, generating data/information of that, and assisting in making an intelligent action by benefiting from collected data. The embodiment of sensors in a building to realize cognitive and adaptive buildings – often, so-called smart buildings – is considered a must.

In residential units, smart thermostats are a ready-to-go appliance which utilizes a motion sensor – mostly passive infrared (PIR) sensors – in order to recognize occupancy. The mismatch between the actual occupancy and the operation schedule of HVAC systems is one of the reasons for energy inefficiency, and it can be managed by this new generation of thermostats. Another benefit is their internet access. It not only allows users to control the appliance remotely but also sends the HVAC operational data into a cloud server.

A Canadian vendor (ecobee) launched a program called Donate Your Data (DYD) that users can share their anonymized data for the sake of research and development in 2015. As an example, researchers could identity certain energy-related patterns and develop prediction models through analyses of such HVAC operational and human behavior data (Huchuk et al., 2019).

The integration of other types of sensors such as infrared cameras, wearable sensors, or even radars has been researched (Jung & Jazizadeh, 2017, 2019). Such efforts will expand the interaction between humans and buildings, touching different dimensions in human dynamics: the number of occupants in a space/thermal zone, physiological responses to the ambient environment, and a physical activity.

Conclusion

Clemson Health Facilities, Baylor College of Medicine and the iCAMP Lab, the Center for Health Design, UA IPWP, GSA, and UA AEDL and its Sensor-Lab are all examples of research agencies, organizations, and interdisciplinary teams which incorporate state-of-the-art technologies in their work on health and wellbeing in the built environment. They play an important role in revealing the potential of using a variety of advanced and emerging technologies including but not limited to wearable devices, environmental sensors, and VR. It gives us much-needed insight on the benefits of these techniques which can aid in determining their overall feasibility and benefits. More research needs to be done, however, on the drawbacks of using a combination of any or all these tools. Since these technologies are rapidly evolving, researchers in the field are faced with the challenge of keeping up with the latest developments and devices, validating them for research purposes, and analyzing enormous amounts of data. All these concerns are discussed in further detail in Chapter 8: Future Directions.

References

The Academy of Neuroscience for Architecture. (2020). Welcome to ANFA. Retrieved from http://www.anfarch.org/

Baylor College of Medicine. (2020). Interdisciplinary consortium on advanced motion performance. Retrieved from https://www.bcm.edu/departments/surgery/research/icamp

The Center for Health Design. (2020). Research coalition. Retrieved from https://www.healthdesign.org/about/volunteers/research-coalition

Clemson University. (2019). Health facilities design and testing. Clemson University, South Carolina. Retrieved from www.clemson.edu/centers-institutes/health-facilities-design-testing/.

Huchuk, B., Sanner, S., & O'Brien, W. (2019). Comparison of machine learning models for occupancy prediction in residential buildings using connected thermostat data. *Building and Environment, 160,* 106177.

Jerdan, S. W., Grindle, M., van Woerden, H. C., & Boulos, M. N. K. (2018). Head-mounted virtual reality and mental health: Critical review of current research. *JMIR Serious Games, 6*(3), e14.

Jung, W., & Jazizadeh, F. (2017). Towards integration of Doppler radar sensors into personalized thermoregulation-based control of HVAC. *Proceedings of the 4th ACM International Conference on Systems for Energy-Efficient Built Environments.* Nov/2017, Article No.: 21, Pages 1–4.

Jung, W., & Jazizadeh, F. (2019). Heat flux sensing for machine-learning-based personal thermal comfort modeling. *Sensors, 19*(17), 3619.

Nikolić, D., Maftei, L., & Whyte, J. (2019). Becoming familiar: How infrastructure engineers begin to use collaborative virtual reality in their interdisciplinary practice. *Journal of Information Technology in Construction (ITcon), 24*(26), 489–508.

Office of the Director of National Intelligence. (2017, September). IARPA launces the "MOSAIC" program to better assess the intelligence community workforce. Retrieved from https://www.dni.gov/index.php/newsroom/press-releases/item/1793-iarpa-launches-mosaic-program-to-better-assess-the-intelligence-community-workforce

The Robert Wood Johnson Foundation. (2018). Leadership for better health. Retrieved from https://www.rwjf.org/

8   Future Directions

Introduction

This book is written at the time of a global pandemic caused by a virus. In December of 2019, a novel coronavirus was identified and traced back to its origins in of Wuhan, China. From its source, it spread rapidly across country lines and was officially named coronavirus disease 2019, which became commonly referred to as COVID-19. Transmission of this virus typically occurs from person-to-person contact with aerosol droplets (Wu et al., 2020). This outbreak was declared a public health emergency of international concern at the end of January 2020 by the World Health Organization's Director-General Ghebreyesus (World Health Organization, 2020). The onset of COVID-19 has fundamentally altered how humans exist in their day-to-day lives as well as revealed how a global pandemic and its subsequent consequences can stimulate rapid innovation in health care.

The COVID-19 crisis has created a massive shift in working and living patterns for people all across the world. We do not fully understand the overall impact on individual health and wellbeing from working remotely, but interim results from extensive global surveys such as the UK's Institute for Employment Studies' (IES) Working from Home Wellbeing Survey (Bevan et al., 2020) indicate an increase in physiological and psychological concerns including an increase in musculoskeletal pain, loss of sleep, deterioration in diet and exercise, and an increase in work-related stress. The fundamental knowledge provided in this book's overarching contents is, therefore, crucial at this time. Employers and employees are now concerned about reentry strategies which include how safe and healthy workplaces can be provided as well as continuously monitored for health and safety. Given this situation, there is an urgent need to conduct rigorous and scientifically accurate human health and built environment research and design followed by real-world applications.

In this concluding chapter, we identify existing knowledge gaps in the field and propose future research directions and built environment design

DOI: 10.4324/9780367814748-12

interventions with a special focus on the global COVID-19 pandemic. It is organized around three basic themes: technologies, research methods and studies, and design methods and systems (Figure 3.2). We suggest directions for human, environmental, and material sensing technology development including Internet of Things (IoT) device developments. Furthermore, smart materials may be linked with actuation and sensing devices to enable real-time responsiveness with human interaction. The connection of intelligent material systems through these smart sensing techniques with the IoT provides a vast territory of unexplored potential in shifting the design of our built environments towards performative actions for human wellbeing (Figure 8.1).

Precedent examples of recent design research on smart materials and intelligent material systems to stay healthy and prevent disease transfer are presented as an overview of concepts in bio-responsive design with emerging materials. Both the potential advantages and the challenges or limitations for bio-responsive systems are discussed. We also discuss the need to further develop core findings that are both generalizable and specific to different design scenarios. We conclude with a forecast on the directions of new systems such as immersive environments, material products, IoT networks, and address the ethics of such possible bio-responsive environments.

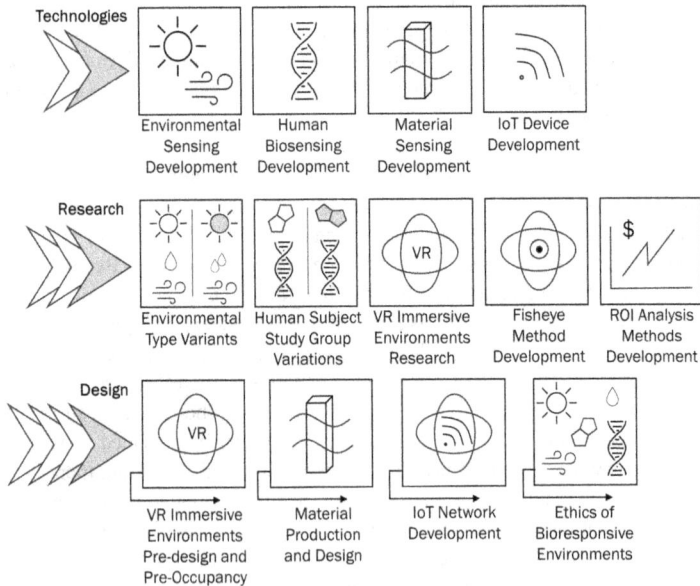

Figure 8.1 Composite Diagram: Bio-responsive Material Systems and Wellbeing.

Technologies: Future Directions

Environmental Sensing Development

While a plethora of environmental sensing devices already exist, the primary developments are occurring in the micro- and nanoscale range. Microbial sensing devices are not widely or readily available and often require laboratory facilities rather than field device deployment. With growing interest in the microbiome of built environments, more microbial sensors are being developed. In addition, the COVID-19 pathogen, severe acute respiratory syndrome coronavirus 2 (SARS-CoV-2), is a recent example of a nanoscale particle that cannot be sensed with current devices. This example demonstrates the challenge of providing substantiated evidence with regard to pathogen transport in airborne and surface contaminant environments and thus the need for developing a wider range of sensing devices. Nanoscale sensors are being developed to assess pathogens at the nanoparticle range (Vishinkin & Haick, 2015).

In conjunction with IoT networks and related smart homes, buildings, and cities, environmental sensors are becoming more rapidly commercialized and deployed on the market for consumer use and accessibility. Some areas of environmental sensing concerns include air and water systems within individual properties, homes, and buildings. Indoor air quality monitoring has a longer track record of commercial and residential use, such as carbon monoxide monitors, but is expanding to incorporate airborne microbes that can serve as indicators of a wider range of allergens and pathogens. Water quality sensing is not typically integrated into buildings and individual properties as the quality of potable water is often seen as the responsibility of the utility and is measured within the main distribution system. Localized premise plumbing sensing devices are still quite expensive and pose challenges to obtaining accurate qualitative measurements under the varying conditions of flow rates and temperatures (Wang et al., 2013). The need for premise plumbing water quality sensing is substantiated from unfortunate scenarios such as Flint, Michigan's 2014–2019 Legionella and lead contaminated water, which exposed between 6,000 and 12,000 children to the related health risks (Centers for Disease Control and Prevention, 2020). Such vast built environment infrastructures and building systems require distributed sensing and ongoing monitoring in addition to strategies and plans for replacement and upgrades to healthier materials and designs.

Human Biosensing Development

Current trends in human biosensing indicate that noninvasive sensors, often either wearable or remote, will soon be able to identify and analyze chemical constituents called analytes in the human body. Sweat, for example, is an extremely informative and important analyte because it contains a remarkable amount of information about one's physiological health and can provide insight into what is needed for personalized medicine. Information such as pH, chloride, glucose, and calcium levels can already be collected from sweat by biosensors, and they have the potential to do more. Interest in flexible and wearable biosensors to measure sweat and other analytes is growing rapidly, and researchers have made important developments in this field. He et al. (2019), for example, have developed a bandage-like biosensor made from a flexible polyester film with a super-hydrophobic silica suspension. The bandage can successfully harvest information about the participant's health which is promising for future biosensors of this nature. Ultimately, the goal for a biosensor like this is to be able to diagnose a number of different types of diseases. Similarly, Jung et al. (2019) proposed to use a heat flux sensor – a sheet of polyimide with differential thermopiles – in wearable devices to capture heat dissipation from the body, regulated by the interaction with ambient environments. Capturing respiratory states remotely using Doppler radar sensors were another attempt to noninvasively quantify human physiological responses to the ambient environments (Jung & Jazizadeh, 2017)

The rapidly spreading coronavirus disease (COVID-19) has made it imperative for labs around the world to accurately test, identify, and treat the virus. The reverse transcription polymerase chain reaction (RT-PCR) has been the primary method for diagnosing the disease so far. It has, however, reported several false-positive and false-negative cases so it is prone to error (Bustin & Nolan, 2004). Fast and accurate testing is imperative during a pandemic because it leads to timely and effective treatment and plans of action to halt the spread. With this goal, Qiu et al. (2020) have combined a dual-functional plasmonic biosensor with a plasmonic photothermal (PPT) effect and localized surface plasmon resonance (LSPR) to reliably detect strains of the coronavirus. This may lead to a sensor that could detect bacteria or viruses that are airborne. These types of fast-acting reliable detection systems are crucial in environments which are dense and crowded such as hospitals and train stations (Qiu et al., 2020). This method may make testing in highly populated areas possible, which can help prevent the spread of the virus.

Another important biosensing innovation has recently been created by engineers at the University of Cincinnati. The research team created a portable testing device which plugs directly into a smartphone. The analyzer is sensitive enough to detect 8 ng/mL and can be used to detect infectious diseases such as coronavirus, malaria, human immunodeficiency virus (HIV), and Lyme disease. This is a significant development at the time of a pandemic, because it can test patients' saliva samples directly at home, thereby eliminating the need to go to a doctor's office. Patients put the single-use plastic chip in their mouth and then plug it into a slot in the device connected to their smartphone. A smartphone app then transmits the results directly to a doctor who analyzes and discusses results with the patient (Ghosh et al., 2020).

Material Sensing Development

Integrated material sensing is less prevalent in the commercial market with the exception of specialized conditions of importance to particular building operations such as hygrothermal monitoring in roof membrane systems over data centers to detect water pooling and leaks. However, with both the onset of COVID-19 and other climate change and health concerns, material sensing developments are becoming more important for human-occupied spaces. Some recent examples of material sensing include carbon nanodots (CNDs) that can be incorporated into cleaning products, which will fluoresce under certain wavelengths of light providing a visual indicator of surface area treatment. This is a useful technique for high-occupancy spaces such as airplane cabins or other high turnover occupancy spaces such as hotel rooms. When these spaces are cleaned, the cleaning efficacy of surfaces can be quickly evaluated and untreated or missed zones can be addressed. Other uses of similar integrated sensing include incorporating nanodot technology into materials to indicate the presence of pathogens, such as SARS-CoV-2, thus allowing for a visual assessment of possible contamination of materials in the built environment.

IoT Device Development

Wearable devices such as smartwatches or other noninvasive sensors connected in real time to the IoT can measure heart rate and skin temperature. As discussed in Chapter 1: Health and wellbeing measures, abnormalities in these measures can be indicative human health issues. Stanford medical researcher, Michael Snyder, is collaborating with Fitbit and Scripps Research to detect early signs of a viral infection through a wearable device via changes in heart rate and skin temperature. Snyder and his team are currently developing an algorithm that can alert users when heart rate or skin temperature or both are elevated – symptoms which indicate that a body is fighting off infection (Armitage, 2020).

Armitage (2020) reported that Snyder's study involves data collection from five different wearable devices using five different algorithms. The participants in the study will keep track of their health status. They are also informed of the importance of contextualizing their situation because not every rise in heart rate is indicative of a viral infection. It is also reported that there are a variety of activities that can cause an increased heart rate such as exercising more or watching a scary movie. This study, however, shows great promise and may be crucial in the current pandemic.

WHOOP is a company which manufactures wrist-worn devices to measure human performance. It is currently collaborating with the Cleveland Clinic and Central Queensland University in Australia in a study in which the wrist-worn device is being worn by hundreds of self-identified COVID-19 patients. By collecting physiological data in the IoT 24 hours a day, seven days a week, university researchers aim to analyze the connection between changes in respiratory rate and COVID-19 symptoms (WHOOP, 2020).

Another study performed by using the WHOOP wearables was centered around sleep. These wearables were worn by 32 participants to track their sleep to determine whether the devices could reliably measure both the quality and the quantity of their sleep. The participants did not have any medical conditions or sleep disorders. They were also asked to self-report their sleep behaviors in daily sleep logs, in which they reported an improvement in nighttime sleep quality. In addition, with this study, WHOOP also became the first wrist-worn wearable device to validate its respiratory rate measuring accuracy during sleep (WHOOP, 2020). This study led the researchers to conclude that smart connected wearable devices could improve sleep quality as well as accurately measure sleep and cardiorespiratory levels (Berryhill et al., 2020). These findings reveal the potential of IoT connected devices to track disease in times of a pandemic.

Research: Future Methods & Studies

Human Subject Study Group Variations

Due to the convenience of hiring students in a university environment, where most research is conducted, a large portion of the studies relies on student or healthy adult populations. For example, the predicted mean vote (PMV) model – widely used in the field of thermal comfort – relied on the data collected form the European average male (ASHRAE Handbook, 2017), which would not represent diversity of individuals, judging thermal environments subjectively. This limitation of the PMV model is thoroughly reviewed by Hoof (2008), indicating that the generalization of human factors possibly misinterprets the thermal environment. This biased data may have skewed our understanding of the influences of indoor environmental quality on humans.

Accordingly, diversifying the demographics of human subjects is needed, even for the established body of knowledge – a validation effort of widely used knowledge/model(s). There could be many factors, including age, gender, and climate. The targeted group of human subjects should be statistically sufficiently gathered to produce meaningful results. It is worth noting that any experiments including human subjects, even surveys, are required to get Institutional Review Board (IRB) approvals. A thorough evaluation of the IRB application is required considering characteristics of subject populations to avoid any risks exposed to the participants.

Another key drive could be the data-sharing culture in this field, which is often costly and time-consuming. Quality data often plays a crucial role in the modeling process on which machine/deep learning techniques, often outperforming the traditional modeling approaches, are often dependent. As an example, similar to the computer vision community, where a large-scale dataset is constructed by the members, the thermal comfort community generated a global scale dataset (Ličina et al., 2018). To facilitate such efforts, a communication platform or community should be formulated and maintained.

Virtual Reality Immersive Environment Research

Virtual reality (VR) has already been used to improve both mental and physical health in different ways, and researchers are currently exploring its usefulness in the COVID-19 pandemic. Nowak et al. (2020) in one VR study used immersive VR to simulate how the flu spreads in relation to an individual's immediate built environment. They gathered participants in ages ranging from 18 to 49 who identified themselves as vaccine avoidant. This meant that the participants were not inclined to get vaccinated for the flu in the current year or the subsequent year. The immersive VR environment was found to create a strong physical sense of the environment for the participants and simultaneously increase the concern they felt for transmitting influenza to other people. Immersive VR was, therefore, found to have the ability to increase the understanding of important concepts related to flu and other diseases, thereby preventing spread and increasing the overall rate of vaccinations (Nowak et al., 2020). This finding has much relevance for today as researchers across the world continue to test various health and built environment interventions and mitigation measures for the pandemic.

Another application of VR is its potential to be a learning platform for health-care professionals. For example, one study investigated the potential and effectiveness of learning for medical students in a virtual world. Students in this study were given the ability to talk to patients and their families about standardized care. This virtual platform was found to be both comfortable and convenient for students. Further, it gave these students more confidence and the ability to practice without the fear of causing any physical harm to a patient since it was all virtual. One criticism of this method was that it was an unfamiliar environment; however, one could conclude that with enough practice, VR could be a useful technique for teaching medical students (Lee et al., 2019).

Mental and physical health are inherently connected. Learning to cope with the fear and anxiety surrounding COVID-19, therefore, is important to survival because these issues could lead to an overall decrease in mental health, changes in eating or sleeping patterns, and chronic health conditions (Centers for Disease Control and Prevention, 2020). Riva and Wiederhold (2020) in a recent study examine how cyberpsychology and VR could help individuals cope with the psychological burden caused by the coronavirus. This subject requires much attention as the psychological distress caused by the coronavirus is long-lasting and cannot be managed easily. Government issued social-distancing and quarantine guidelines can negatively impact one's everyday experiences and health. As technological advances in VR increase, so does its cost-effectiveness and, in turn, the ability to make it readily available to the public. Since immersive 360-degree videos can illicit specific emotions and can help improve cognitive processes, these researchers suggest using VR for a week, two or more times a day, as an emotional regulation tool. They also find that VR can provide individuals with a safe place to escape in an environment where it is difficult to redirect emotional strain. VR, therefore, is a useful tool for individuals to reflect on their identity and fight rumination in times like today that are inherently stressful to society (Riva & Wiederhold, 2020).

Fisheye Method Development

The fisheye analysis method is not often utilized in built environment research and design and most frequently accessed for vegetation and agriculture studies. Some contemporary examples of the use of fisheye analysis include a study by the architecture firm Kieran Timberlake for a campus planning project at the University of Washington. In this study, a detailed digital model of an existing natural ecology was documented to assess the potential impacts of proposed construction activities. The research team was able to analyze the effective thermal comfort of the microclimate based on fisheye methods of the tree canopies, which also enabled them to calculate rain and stormwater absorption in the exposed ground surface area. All together this information established a quantifiable understanding of the local ecosystem contribution to carbon absorption, stormwater management, and potential energy savings through tree shading. This is a good example of how the fisheye method might be accessed for providing more comprehensive assessment of built environment conditions on human wellbeing aspects, such as thermal comfort and other sensory phenomena.

Return on Investment Analysis Methods Development

As employees return to their workplaces in the current and post-COVID-19 situation, companies are brainstorming ways to minimize risk to people and stay operational at the same time. Employers must now consider not only current pandemic conditions but also post-pandemic conditions, and future new pandemics. This effort will also lead to new return on investment (ROI) methods. In order to be effective, the ROI plan and budget should include providing evidence-based optimal, as well as over-and-above building standards ranges, for ventilation, air quality, thermal health, moisture, dusts and pests, safety and security, water quality, noise, and lighting and views – all of which constitute the foundations of healthy building as per Allen and Macomber (2020). Further, it should include continuous sensing and monitoring systems for these building systems. These systems should display and record real-time actual measures versus optimum levels of these environmental attributes and communicate safety warnings. As discussed in previous chapters, these monitoring technologies would not only lead to minimizing risk but also improve employee performance. Companies that do not keep up with such technological innovations may unfortunately find themselves to be unprepared now, as well as in the future. One strategy may be to appoint a key point person such as a facilities manager, assisted by a task force to keep track of rapidly developing innovative health and safety solutions and implement them effectively.

Design: Future Methods & Systems

VR Immersive Environments Predesign and Preoccupancy

VR immersive environments allow stakeholders and end users to experience built environments at a predesign or preoccupancy stages, that is, before they have actually been built or occupied. Using VR in this phase has the potential to assess early proposals, avoid costly errors, and provide solutions that are more user-centric. For example, VR health-care educational environments could improve first-person active learning by allowing users to interact with their environments before they are actually built. Besides simulating rooms and workflow, they are useful for a variety of forms of education ranging from three-dimensional anatomical models to creating a patient avatar that students can interact with (Kyaw et al., 2019). While the research surrounding virtual patients (VPs) is limited, there is still potential to use them to simulate useful virtual learning environments. Further research is needed to simulate the wide range of symptoms patients may experience to ensure a broader use for the students while still maintaining a consistent level of education (Combs & Combs, 2019). Once there is more information on how VR influences treatment outcomes as well as satisfaction of medical professionals and patients, it may prove to be a cost-effective method to positively influence overall clinical practice (Kyaw et al., 2019) and create built environments for health care and other fields, based on actual user feedback at the predesign stage.

Material Production and Design

In the most recent years, there has been a push to move to healthy building materials, which largely focuses on the removal of chemical contaminants for building products. One of the most noteworthy and publicized events early in this history that provided momentum to this movement was the Federal

Emergency Management Agency (FEMA)'s trailers that were distributed to residents who lost their homes in Hurricane Katrina in New Orleans, Louisiana, in 2005. After living in the units, residents complained of various health ailments, including flu-like symptoms, and the trailers were found to have high levels of formaldehyde, a toxic carcinogen, in the indoor air. On closer inspection, the trailers were found to have had been built with pressed wood and glues emitting high levels of the chemical (Verderber, 2008). Consequently, the US federal government made changes to the design and materials used in these emergency housing structures.

There are a number of organizations working to reduce harmful chemicals and increase transparency in the building industry. Once such collective is the Healthy Building Network (HBN) which is an organization of engineers, researchers, scientists, and educators using research and policy, data tools, and education to inform and protect the public (HBN, 2023). This organization through the Health Product Declaration Collaborative (HPDC) has been instrumental in pushing the Leadership in Energy and Environmental Design (LEED) to adopt health-based materials credits. The HPDC collects manufacture's product material information in disclosures. This information can be accessed by the construction industry to allow builders to choose greener products.

Biogenic design is the use of natural materials with a focus on materials that are carbon sequestering or low carbon emitting. These are largely renewable, low-energy alternatives with options for reuse that promote a sustainable, circular closed loop system and can include products composted of yeast, bacteria, algae, chitin, and hemp. One example is the rootlike structure of fungus known as mycelium, whose fibers can be used in various aspects of buildings including structural materials and insulation (Attias et al., 2019). These materials are low cost, low energy, light in weight, and biodegradable. Mycelium has moved into the commercial space where various products including walls and floors can be purchased in lieu of other less sustainable options (Mogu, 2022).

IoT Network Developments

The expansion of the IoT network for built environment and human health is rapidly occurring. Numerous sensing devices are being connected with apps and mobile devices, and sometimes, this information and data are collected into larger-scale information databases and networks. One example of a multifunctional IoT device is the Scanning MeAn Radiant Temperature (SMART) sensing technology produced at the Cooling and Heating for Architecturally Optimized Systems (CHAOS) lab at Princeton University's Andlinger Center for Energy and the Environment (Princeton C.H.A.O.S Laboratory, n.d.). The SMART sensor incorporates a three-dimensional representation of the surfaces of a space and provides the radiant thermal value (reradiation or emissivity) of each source with an embedded rotating infrared sensor platform. The SMART sensor is then able to make a calculation of the effective thermal comfort at the location of the sensing device as well as discover sources of pollution. When connected to building information system networks, the SMART devices can enable the optimization of energy performance for human thermal comfort and improve air quality. Building management systems of the future will integrate more information, including biometrics of its occupants and microbial sensing of interior biomes, for more advanced knowledge about the health of buildings.

Ethics of Bio-responsive Environments

The advancements and increasing adoption of biosensing technologies (wearable and remote) in the built environment raise a concern of privacy. Specifically, in the pathway for automated building systems, individuals' physiological/physical/psychological data is required for accurate prediction and control. This calls for systematic data privacy and management, which start from ethical use of such data. In recent years, a number of unethical attempts across disciplines drew attention from the public. Such unethical acts possibly create harm to the persons who were willing to share their private data for analyses and use. In order to prevent this unwanted result from happening, a variety of technological barriers, including data encryption methods, can be built within systems. Another example is to manage individual's identifiable data, as often suggested by the IRB. In the end, building systems can decentralize and remove individual identities for operation.

Conclusions

As countries across the globe continue to fight the COVID-19 pandemic, we anticipate all the new techniques and methods to measure the impact of the built environment on health, wellbeing, and performance described in this book, and beyond, to play a critical role in understanding and developing new design interventions and strategies to counter disease transmission. Additionally, lockdown, home isolation, and social distancing measures have increased our awareness of how our surrounding environments influence our wellbeing. The three parts of this book – fundamentals, methods, and applications – provide both the foundational knowledge and fundamentals for characterizing human health and wellbeing in the built environment as well as emerging trends and design research methods for innovations in this field. We hope to inspire researchers, educators, and students in universities, researchers and professionals in the built environment industry and integrative medicine, human resource professionals, facilities managers, developers, building owners, and real estate professionals, and design and build environments that optimize the health, wellbeing, and performance of the workforce. As both employers and employees ponder ways to create safe work environments for reentry or healthy and comfortable remote work environments, this information is of vital importance. In addition, we hope that the research methodologies, technical innovations, and case studies, discussed in this book, will make an impact on government agencies and organizations who are invested in research, setting standards, and shaping policy in health and built environment.

References

Allen, J. G., & Macomber, J. D. (2020, April). What makes an office building "healthy"? *Harvard Business Review*. Retrieved from https://hbr.org/2020/04/what-makes-an-office-building-healthy

American Society of Heating, Refrigerating, and Air-conditioning Engineers (ASHRAE). (2017). ASHRAE Handbook – Fundamentals – Chapter 9. Thermal comfort. ASHRAE Inc.

Armitage, H. (2020, April 14). Stanford medicine scientists hope to use data from wearable devices to predict illness, including COVID-19. Retrieved from https://med.stanford.edu/news/all-news/2020/04/wearable-devices-for-predicting-illness-.html

Attias, M., Danai, O., Tarazi, E., Pereman I., & Grobman, Y. J. (2019) Implementing bio-design tools to develop mycelium-based products. *The Design Journal*, *22*(Suppl. 1), 1647–1657. https://doi.org/10.1080/14606925.2019.1594997

Berryhill, S., Morton, C. J., Dean, A., Berryhill, A., Provencio-Dean, N., Patel, S. I., ... & Krishnan, J. A. (2020). Effect of wearables on sleep in healthy individuals: A randomized cross-over trial and validation study. *Journal of Clinical Sleep Medicine*, jcsm-8356. J Clin Sleep Med 2020 May 15;16(5):775–783. doi: 10.5664/jcsm.8356. Epub 2020 Feb 11.

Bevan, S., Mason, B., & Bajorek, Z. (2020). Homeworker wellbeing survey: Interim results. Institute from Employment Studies (IES), UK. Retrieved from https://www.employment-studies.co.uk/resource/ies-working-home-wellbeing-survey

Bustin, S., & Nolan, T. (2004). Pitfalls of quantitative real-time reverse-transcription polymerase chain reaction. Journal of Biomolecular Techniques, 15(3), 155–166.

Centers for Diseases Control and Prevention. (2020a). Flint water crisis. Retrieved from https://www.cdc.gov/nceh/casper/pdf-html/flint_water_crisis_pdf.html

Centers for Diseases Control and Prevention. (2020b). Mental health and coping during COVID-19. Retrieved from https://www.cdc.gov/coronavirus/2019-ncov/daily-life-coping/managing-stress-anxiety.html

Combs, C Donald, and P Ford Combs. "Emerging Roles of Virtual Patients in the Age of AI." *AMA journal of ethics* vol. 21,2 E153–159. 1 Feb. 2019, doi:10.1001/amajethics.2019.153

He, X., Xu, T., Gu, Z., Gao, W., Xu, L. P., Pan, T., & Zhang, X. (2019). Flexible and super-wettable bands as a platform toward sweat sampling and sensing. *Analytical Chemistry*, *91*(7), 4296–4300.

Ghosh, S., Aggarwal, K., Vinitha, T. U., Nguyen, T., Han, J., & Ahn, C. H. (2020). A new microchannel capillary flow assay (MCFA) platform with lyophilized chemiluminescence reagents for a smartphone-based POCT detecting malaria. *Microsystems & Nanoengineering*, *6*(1), 1–18.

Healthy Building Network (HBN). (2023). Building a healthy world. Retrieved from https://healthybuilding.net/about

Hoof, v. (2008). Forty years of Fanger's model of thermal comfort: Comfort for all? *Indoor*, *18*(3), 182–201.

Jung, W., & Jazizadeh, F. (2017). Towards integration of Doppler radar sensors into personalized thermoregulation-based control of HVAC. Proceedings of the 4th ACM

International Conference on Systems for Energy-Efficient Built Environments. Nov/2017, Article No.: 21, Pages 1–4.

Jung, W., Jazizadeh, F., & Diller, T. (2019). Heat Flux sensing for machine-learning-based personal thermal comfort modeling. *Sensors, 19*(17), 3691.

Kyaw, B. M., Saxena, N., Posadzki, P., Vseteckova, J., Nikolaou, C. K., George, P. P., … & Car, L. T. (2019). Virtual reality for health professions education: Systematic review and meta-analysis by the Digital Health Education collaboration. *Journal of Medical Internet Research, 21*(1), e12959.

Lee, A. L., DeBest, M., Koeniger-Donohue, R., Strowman, S. R., & Mitchell, S. E. (2019). The feasibility and acceptability of using virtual world technology for interprofessional education in palliative care: A mixed methods study. *Journal of Interprofessional Care*, 1–11. J Interprof Care 2020 Jul-Aug;34(4):461–471. doi: 10.1080/13561820.2019.1643832. Epub 2019 Aug 21.

Ličina, V., Cheung, T., & Zhang, H., et al. (2018). Development of the ASHRAE Global thermal comfort Database II. *Buidling and Environment, 142*, 502–512.

Mogu. (2022). *Mycelium.* Retrieved from https://mogu.bio/about/mycelium-technology/

Nowak, G. J., Evans, N. J., Wojdynski, B. W., Ahn, S. J. G., Len-Rios, M. E., Carera, K., … & McFalls, D. (2020). Using immersive virtual reality to improve the beliefs and intentions of influenza vaccine avoidant 18-to-49-year-olds: Considerations, effects, and lessons learned. *Vaccine, 38*(5), 1225–1233.

Princeton C.H.A.O.S. Laboratory. n.d. S.M.A.R.T. SENSOR. Retrieved from https://chaos.princeton.edu/outputs/smart-sensor/

Qiu, G., Gai, Z., Tao, Y., Schmitt, J., Kullak-Ublick, G. A., & Wang, J. (2020). Dual-functional plasmonic photothermal biosensors for highly accurate severe acute respiratory syndrome Coronavirus 2 detection. *ACS Nano* 2020 May 26;14(5):5268–5277. doi: 10.1021/acsnano.0c02439. Epub 2020 Apr 13.

Riva, G., & Wiederhold, B. K. (2020). How cyberpsychology and virtual reality can help us to overcome the psychological burden of Coronavirus. Editorial Cyberpsychol Behav Soc Netw. 2020 May;23(5):277–279. doi: 10.1089/cyber.2020.29183. gri Epub 2020 Apr 17.

Verderber, S. (2008). Emergency housing in the aftermath of Hurricane Katrina: An assessment of the FEMA travel trailer program. *Journal of Housing and the Built Environment, 23*, 367–381. https://doi.org/10.1007/s10901-008-9124-y

Vishinkin, R., & Haick, H. (2015). Nanoscale sensor technologies for disease detection via volatolomics. *Small, 11*(46), 6142–6164.

Wang, H., Edwards, M., Falkinham, J., & Pruden, A. (2013). Probiotic approach to pathogen control in premise plumbing systems? A review. *Environmental Science & Technology, 47*(18), 10117–10128.

WHOOP (2020, April 1). WHOOP investigating respiratory rate pattern and relationship with COVID-19 symptoms. Retrieved from https://www.prnewswire.com/news-releases/whoop-investigating-respiratory-rate-pattern-and-relationship-with-covid-19-symptoms-301033339.html

World Health Organization. (2020, January 30). Coronavirus disease (COVID-19) - events as they happen. Retrieved from https://www.who.int/emergencies/diseases/novel-coronavirus-2019/events-as-they-happen

Wu, Y. C., Chen, C. S., & Chan, Y. J. (2020). The outbreak of COVID-19: An overview. *Journal of the Chinese Medical Association, 83*(3), 217. https://kierantimberlake.com/page/mapping-surveying

Index

Note: *Italic* page numbers refer to figures.

For Product Safety Concerns and Information please contact our EU
representative GPSR@taylorandfrancis.com
Taylor & Francis Verlag GmbH, Kaufingerstraße 24, 80331 München, Germany

www.ingramcontent.com/pod-product-compliance
Lightning Source LLC
Chambersburg PA
CBHW061330220326
41599CB00026B/5118

9 7 8 1 0 3 2 7 4 6 1 2 8